Heart Advice
for Death and Dying

Heart Advice
for Death and Dying

Lama Zopa Rinpoche
with Audio Course by Kathleen McDonald

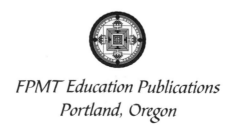

FPMT Education Publications
Portland, Oregon

FPMT Inc.
1632 SE 11th Avenue
Portland, OR 97214 USA
www.fpmt.org

ISBN-13: 978-0-9729028-2-3

Cover design by Lynn Shwadchuck. Cover photo of Medicine Buddha thangka taken from the stock of the FPMT Foundation Store taken by Noah Grunnell.
© FPMT Inc.

Line drawings of Milarepa, Shakyamuni Buddha, Thousand-arm Chenrezig, and Four-arm Chenrezig © Robert Beer. Used with permission.

Line drawings of the Medicine Buddhas © Andy Weber. Used with permission.

Set in Goudy Old Style 12./15 and BiblScrT.

Printed in the USA on 30% PCW recycled paper, FSC Certified.

Contents

PREFACE   7

INTRODUCTION   11
  by Kathleen McDonald

TEACHINGS BY LAMA ZOPA RINPOCHE   31
Impermanence and Death   33
  Meditation: Life is Finishing Quickly   45

The Nine-Point Meditation on Death   49

The Process of Dying   65

Preparing for Death   73

Practicing the Five Powers   83
  Meditation: Tonglen   117

Caring for the Dying and the Dead   123

Essential Activities at the Death Time   131

Medicine Buddha Sadhana   135
  The Benefits of Medicine Buddha Practice 137
  The Medicine Buddha Sadhana   141

Mantras to Benefit the Dying and Dead   149

Helpful Resources   151

Biographies   155

Glossary   157

Notes   167

Index   171

Consciousness doesn't just cease at the time of death. It is not like a lamp that goes out when the fuel is finished. The body and mind are totally separate; they are two different phenomena.
                                        - Lama Zopa Rinpoche

PREFACE

All spiritual traditions provide teachings on death and how to live our lives to obtain the best possible result after death. In our busy modern lives, we may not give much thought to our deaths, and indeed, we may be uncomfortable even thinking about death. We feel it is too depressing and fear that thinking about death will make us sad; we think it will take all the joy out of living. However, when we actively think about death and prepare for our own deaths, the opposite happens – we actually find peace, fulfillment, and happiness in our current lives, and our fear of death disappears.

The Tibetan Buddhist tradition gives extensive teachings on death from every conceivable angle. Whether you want to know how the death process occurs, what happens after death, how to prepare for death, or how to make our lives most meaningful, Tibetan Buddhism has answers.

Recently, the Tibetan Buddhist master Lama Zopa Rinpoche asked that his teachings on death and dying be made available so that all students – beginners to advanced – have access to this most essential advice for this crucial time of transition from one life to the next. In response to this request, many Dharma centers under the care of Lama Zopa Rinpoche began teaching courses on death, and we at Rinpoche's organization, the Foundation for the Preservation of the Mahayana Tradition (FPMT), developed this book and audio course, as well as a program offered in FPMT Dharma centers around the world.

Heart Advice for Death and Dying contains Lama Zopa Rinpoche's essential advice for the time of death and for finding the deepest fulfillment in life. Whether you are taking this class at an FPMT

Dharma center or participating in the audio course that accompanies this book, you will come away with a plethora of practical advice, meditation practices to prepare for your own death (starting now!), knowledge of the heart practices for the time of death, and the working knowledge you need to assist others who are dying or who have died. This course may be enjoyed by students at any level; neither the course nor this book are intended for new students alone.

The MP3 disc that accompanies this book contains an audio course consisting of eleven hours of exquisite teachings and meditations on death led by Kathleen McDonald (Venerable Sangye Khadro). It also contains course handouts, the meditations, and a list of suggested further reading. You may listen to the teachings at home, while driving or traveling, while sitting in the park, or wherever one likes! The meditations included in this book and in the course are essential for taking these teachings into your heart and using them to transform your life.

This book begins with an introduction by Kathleen McDonald, which is followed by the teachings of Lama Zopa Rinpoche. These teachings are the reading material for the course, and may also stand alone as profound teachings on the subject of death.

This book also contains a short Medicine Buddha practice that may be done to benefit those who are dying or who have died, as well as a precious mantra sheet that may be placed on the body of those who have died to bring them the most benefit. The many other practices, mantras, and prayers mentioned in this book may be found in a companion volume, *Heart Practices for Death and Dying*, which is available from FPMT at www.fpmt.org/shop.

If you find this book and audio course useful, you may also be interested in other educational offerings from FPMT. We offer an extensive array of study programs in our centers and as homestudy or correspondence courses, starting with short introductory courses such as Meditation 101 and Buddhism in a Nutshell; Discovering Buddhism, the foundational two-year course on the stages of the path to enlightenment, as well as Foundation of

Buddhist Thought, which is taught through our London center; and advanced study of philosophical texts in the Basic Program, Maitripa College, and the seven-year Masters Program. More information is available at www.fpmt.org/education. Please join us!

Many people contributed to the creation of this book and course. We extend our deepest thanks to Venerable Tenzin Chogkyi for creating the general outline of the course, to the creators and editors of the Discovering Buddhism program, to the Lama Yeshe Wisdom Archive (www.lamayeshe.com) for providing the glossary of this book, and for their precious work archiving and making the teachings of Lama Thubten Yeshe and Lama Zopa Rinpoche available. And thanks to Venerable Constance Miller and Sherry Tillery for their generous time in providing feedback.

We especially thank Kathleen McDonald for her beautiful teachings and for sharing her time and considerable experience with us. And from the bottom of our hearts we thank Lama Zopa Rinpoche, who out of his great compassion and inconceivable kindness, has made these essential heart instructions available for the benefit of all. We hope this book and audio course bring everlasting happiness to sentient beings everywhere.

Gyalten Mindrol
FPMT International Office
Portland, Oregon, USA
October 2008

*The Buddha told his listeners not to blindly be-
lieve what was written in a sacred book or spoken
by a holy person, including himself. He said we
should use our intelligence to check things out for
ourselves and determine what is true and false,
right and wrong.*

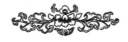

INTRODUCTION

by Kathleen McDonald

I am writing this introduction a few weeks after the death of my mother. Her death was a difficult experience for me - it's always painful losing someone you love, someone important in your life – but it was also beautiful and inspiring. My mother was diagnosed with advanced-stage cancer in early December and died at home three weeks later. I feel very fortunate that I could stay with her during those last weeks of her life, until her last breath. She was completely accepting of her illness and impending death, was not unhappy or afraid, and instead was peaceful, loving and caring towards others, even cheerful. She had no pain, physical or mental, right up to the end.

I believe her life and death were an illustration of the main theme of this book, that how we die depends on how we live. If we wish to be peaceful and positive at the time of death, we need to develop and live those qualities as much as we can in our life. My mother's ability to be serene, content and positive as she neared death was the result of a life of faith, gratitude, optimism, goodness, and kindness to others.

The subject of death makes a lot of people uneasy. They don't like to think, talk, or hear about death. If something related to death comes up in a conversation, there is an uncomfortable silence, then we quickly change the subject. Part of the problem is lack of knowledge. We just don't know much about death, what to do about it, how to prepare for it. We don't have courses on "Death Management" at our local community college or adult-education center.

This problem has been somewhat remedied over the last forty years or so, thanks to the hospice movement and writers such as Elisabeth Kübler-Ross and Stephen Levine. Death and dying have come out of the shadows and are now more acceptable topics of conversation, but there is still a long way to go.

Death is a very important subject in Buddhism. There is a great deal of information on what death is all about, why it happens, how we can prepare for our own death, and how we can help others who are dying. In this book, Lama Zopa Rinpoche shares with us the wisdom of the Tibetan Buddhist tradition on this subject. Some readers may not be familiar with Buddhism, and particularly Tibetan Buddhism, so in this introduction I will explain some basic Buddhist ideas about life, death, and what happens after death.

The Buddhist World View

There are different ideas about where we come from, why we are here, and what happens to us when we die. Some people believe in a creator who gave us life, intelligence, free will, and a soul that will live forever after death. Other people believe that we are nothing more than a collection of biological substances and processes, and that our life simply ceases when we die, like a flame going out.

The Buddhist explanation is that we are part of a universe in which there are myriad worlds and living beings, continuously coming into existence and going out of existence. This situation is known as samsara, or cyclic existence. There is no beginning to this process and no creator. The driving force behind everything that happens – in the universe as well as in our individual lives – is karma, the law of cause and effect. More will be said about this later, but in brief, karma means that we experience the results or effects of our actions. It means that we are the creators of our own experiences.

Cyclic existence is not a perfect, delightful situation, but rather an imperfect, unsatisfactory one. We are born, age, and die again and again. Between each birth and death, we experience many difficulties: sickness, loss, relationship problems, disappointment, depression, irritation, worries, and so on. Of course, not all of our experiences are bad – we have pleasant ones as well, but even those are unsatisfying. They don't completely free us from our problems, and they don't last.

This may sound depressing, and in fact Buddhism is often accused of being pessimistic, but the Buddha did not teach only about problems and suffering; he also explained that there is an alternative to samsara: nirvana, or liberation, the state of perfect peace, bliss, and freedom from all problems. Moreover, there is the state of complete enlightenment, or Buddhahood, the attainment of which enables us to be of benefit to all beings throughout space. These states are attainable by each and every one of us. In fact, according to Buddhism, that is the ultimate purpose of our life: striving to attain either nirvana – self-liberation from the cycle of birth and death – or enlightenment, in order to help all beings become free. And we don't have to wait until reaching nirvana or enlightenment for things to improve. As we progress along the spiritual path, we will experience less suffering and more happiness, and our ability to benefit others will also increase.

The Buddha told his listeners not to blindly believe what was written in a sacred book or spoken by a holy person, including himself. He said we should use our intelligence to check things out for ourselves and determine what is true and false, right and wrong. And we *can* know what is true. Our minds have unlimited potential; the very nature of the mind is clear, pure, and endowed with many positive qualities. This clarity and purity is only temporarily clouded by obstructing factors such as delusions and karma, the very things that keep us stuck in samsara. These factors can be eliminated gradually through spiritual practice, so that the pure, clear "Buddha-nature" of our minds can become manifest. Once we become enlightened, we will experience the true nature of all things in a direct and unmistaken way.

The attainment of enlightenment does not happen instantly. It happens gradually over time, as we engage in spiritual practice. The spiritual path is a process, and one of the first steps in this process is acknowledging the reality of impermanence and death.

The Importance of Remembering Impermanence and Death

The Buddha frequently spoke about impermanence: that things are not fixed and static, but transitory, changing moment by moment. This is true of people and other living beings, everything in nature, and all human creations. Also, all these things will not last forever, but will inevitably die or go out of existence. The Buddha said:

> All collections end up running out,
> The high end up falling,
> Meeting ends in separation,
> Living ends in death.

Buddha also recommended that we accept, contemplate, and remain aware of impermanence and death, rather than denying or avoiding this reality. He said:

> Of all ploughing, ploughing in the autumn is supreme.
> Of all footprints, the elephant's is supreme.
> Of all perceptions, remembering death and impermanence
>   is supreme.

Why do we need to remember impermanence and death? Let's look at what can happen if we don't remember it. We may feel as though we will live forever and that we don't have to prepare for death. Or we may think that the only purpose in life is to enjoy ourselves as much as possible. With such attitudes, we may be careless about what we do, and fail to do what is really important with our life. We may act in ways that are selfish, dishonest, or even cruel. Such a life will be unsatisfying and even harmful to both ourselves and others, and in the end we may die with regret and fear.

On the other hand, awareness of the transitory nature of everything leads us to be careful about what we do, and stimulates positive attitudes and behavior. People who have near-death experiences confirm this. These are people who have a close encounter with death, but then have a second chance at life. They come back with a strong sense of the importance of being loving and caring towards others, of the insignificance of materialistic pursuits, and of having a spiritual dimension in their life.

We don't have to have a near-death experience to realize these important truths; being consistently mindful of impermanence and death will have the same effect.

Death is Not the End of Everything

According to Buddhism, our present life is just one in a series of lives that stretch far back into the past, and will continue far into the future, until we attain liberation or enlightenment. A person is a combination of body and mind. The body consists of all the physical aspects of our being: skin, bones, blood, organs, cells, atoms, and so forth. The mind, on the other hand, is non-physical; it is not made of atoms, cells, or any material substance. The mind consists of all of our conscious experiences: thoughts, emotions, perceptions, memories, dreams, fantasies, and so on. It is not a fixed, static phenomenon, but an ever-changing stream of experiences. We can see this for ourselves by simply observing our inner world. One moment there's a happy thought or feeling, the next moment an unhappy one. We are loving at one moment, angry at another. Memories of the past and fantasies of the future flow in and out amidst perceptions of the present moment. The mind is never the same from one moment to the next.

While we are alive, our body and mind have an interdependent relationship: what happens in our minds affects our bodies, and vice-versa. This is confirmed by recent research on the effects of people's emotions on their health and lifespan. But the mind-body relationship is transient and ends with death. Death is the point at which the mind separates from the body. The body is left behind to be buried or cremated, and the mind, which never dies, travels on to connect with a new body and begin a new life. So death is not a final end, but rather a gateway to another life. However, what passes from this life to the next is not a fixed, personal identity or soul, but rather the impersonal, ever-changing mind stream, carrying with it imprints of all we have done in our life. These imprints determine the experiences we will have in the future.

Normally, a person's mind does not separate from the body as soon as they stop breathing, but later, sometimes hours or even days afterwards. Tibetan Buddhism contains an explanation of the process of dying, which takes place in eight stages. Lama Zopa Rinpoche gives a brief description of this process in Chapter 3, and you can check the recommended reading list for further information.

Rebirth also does not usually occur right away, but could take up to seven weeks, or forty-nine days. The period between death and the next birth is known as the bardo, or intermediate state. Again, this topic is only briefly mentioned in this book, so check the recommended reading list if you would like to learn more about it.

Karma

The circumstances of our next life – the place of birth, our parents, whether we are healthy or unhealthy, rich or poor, clever or dull, and all the experiences we will have – are not a matter of choice, as some people think, but are the results of what we did in this life as well as our previous lives. This is karma. Karma is a Sanskrit word that literally means "action." Each time we do an action, an imprint is left on our minds that will bring results in the future when the right conditions come together.

Karma can be divided into actions of body, speech and mind. We create karma with our physical actions, our words, and even with our thoughts. Also, in a general way, karma can be divided into positive and negative. The main factor that determines whether an action is positive or negative is the motivation behind it. We create positive karma when we act with the wish to help and not harm others, and with our minds free of delusions such as anger and attachment. The future results of such actions will be positive experiences such as good health, being treated kindly by others, having enough of what we need, and so on. On the other hand, when we are motivated by a negative attitude such as anger or attachment, and do actions such as hurting someone, stealing, or being dishonest, we create negative karma. Negative karma is the cause of unpleasant experiences in the future, such as health problems, poverty, failure, or being treated badly by others.

Lama Thubten Yeshe used to say that we don't have to wait until our next life to observe how karma works. Even in this life, or in one day, we can see that our attitudes and behavior at one point in time affect our experiences at a later point. If we wake up in a bad mood – unhappy about our life, our job, the world, the kind of person we are – and go to work in such a mental state, it is pretty definite that we will have problems that day. On the other hand, if we start our day with a positive mental state – happy with ourselves, our life, and the people around us – most of our experiences that day will be pleasant and satisfying.

Karma is not something fixed, like words carved in stone; just because we have done something negative doesn't mean we will necessarily have to suffer. We can purify our negative karma and not have to experience its suffering results. Karmic purification is a psychological process involving four steps:

1. Feeling regret for what we have done;
2. Relying upon helpful objects of refuge, such as the Buddha or another higher power who is wise, compassionate, and forgiving, as well as on cultivating positive attitudes such as love and compassion;
3. Doing something positive as a remedy to the negative action;
4. Resolving to refrain from repeating the action in the future.

There is no karma that cannot be purified by using these four, which are known as the four opponent powers.

Understanding and accepting karma means taking responsibility. We realize that we are the creators of our experiences. We can't blame anyone for our problems, and we can't expect that someone else can make us happy. This understanding is crucial for our present life: if we want happiness and positive experiences, we must create the right causes; and if we don't want unhappiness and bad experiences, we must avoid creating the causes for those.

Understanding karma is also essential when we look ahead to the end of our life and what will happen afterwards. The experiences we will have as we are dying and afterwards are determined by our actions in this life. A positive, loving life leads to good experiences at death and in the next life, while a selfish, destructive life leads to negative experiences at death and in the next life.

Aside from karma, another crucial factor that determines our experiences in the next life is the state of mind we have at death. The reason for this is that most of us will arrive at the end of our lives with a vast collection of both positive and negative karma. Which of these karmic imprints will be the cause of our next life? That is determined by our state of mind as we die. A positive state of mind – accepting, calm, and loving – will activate one of our positive karmic imprints and propel us to a fortunate rebirth. A negative state of mind – non-accepting, clinging to people or possessions, or angry at what is happening to us – will activate one of our negative karma imprints, propelling our minds to unfortunate rebirths.

From the Buddhist point of view, this is the main reason for aspiring to die with a positive state of mind. It's not only for our deaths to be pleasant rather than horrible; it's so that where we go and what we experience after death will be positive. For spiritual practitioners, the real goal is being born in a situation where we will meet spiritual teachers and teachings, and be able to continue following the spiritual path to the higher states of liberation and enlightenment.

The Precious Human Life

According to Buddhism, there are different situations where we could be born after we die. Some of these are fortunate, resulting from positive karma; they include the human, sura (demigod), and asura (god) realms. Others are unfortunate, the result of negative karma: the animal, hungry ghost, and hell realms. Of all places of rebirth, the best from the point of view of spiritual practice is the human realm. The reason for this is that as human beings we have just the right amount of difficulties to be able to recognize the unsatisfactory situation we are in as unenlightened beings and to aspire to be free from it, but we are not so overwhelmed by problems that we are unable to do anything constructive. Most of the beings in the other realms either have too much suffering or too much pleasure to be able to develop these attitudes.

But even in the human realm, not everyone is in the best situation for spiritual practice, so Buddhism speaks of the 'precious human rebirth.' This is a particular kind of human life in which we have all the ideal internal and external conditions in which to follow a spiritual path that leads out of suffering and dissatisfaction, to genuine peace, happiness and enlightenment. These conditions include having access to spiritual teachers and teachings that show the path to enlightenment, having faith in these teachings, wanting to learn and practice them, and being supported in our practice by caring family and/or friends.

A precious human rebirth does not come about by chance; it is the result of creating certain causes. The main cause of such a life is living ethically, which means refraining from harmful actions such as killing, stealing, lying, and so on. Other important causes are generosity, patience, being energetic about doing positive actions, and making prayers for such a rebirth. This means that if we have a precious human rebirth now, we must have created these causes in our past lives. And if we want such a rebirth next time, we need to create these causes now, in this life.

The usual way in which the precious human rebirth is discussed in the Buddhist teachings is in terms of recognizing that we are extremely fortunate to have such a life. This is because of the many meaningful and beneficial things we can do with this life, for ourselves and others, now and in the future. The precious human rebirth is also rare and difficult to obtain, so while we have this opportunity, before it ends, we need to use it wisely and carefully.

Bodhichitta - the Aspiration to Attain Enlightenment

The most meaningful and beneficial thing we can do with our precious human life is to develop our Buddha nature, our potential for enlightenment. Why is this? Because the most meaningful work of all is benefiting others. And until we are enlightened, our ability to help others is limited. We can see this for ourselves. Sometimes we feel lazy or caught up in self-concern and we are not interested in helping others. Even when we do feel like helping others, we may quickly lose interest or get burned out, and may even become angry if the people we are helping don't cooperate with us. Because we lack wisdom, we sometimes make mistakes in the things we do to help, making things worse rather than better.

Enlightened beings never have such problems. They have inexhaustible, unconditional love and compassion for all beings without exception. Their wisdom is perfect - they always know the most skillful way to help each individual. They never run out of energy. They are free of their own needs, so they never get tired or burned out; they don't even need holidays or coffee breaks!

Enlightenment is a state we can all attain. But we first need to develop bodhichitta, the aspiration to attain enlightenment in order to help all beings. With this motivation, everything we do - even ordinary actions like eating, sleeping and working - becomes a cause for enlightenment. Lama Zopa Rinpoche says that the best attitude we can have as we die is that of bodhichitta. Therefore, generating bodhichitta and directing our energy towards enlightenment is the best way to use our human life and our death.

But this does not mean that we cannot help others until we are enlightened. Generating and practicing bodhichitta also means doing whatever we can to help others now, and it adds another dimension to such actions. For example, when we give food to a homeless person or help our neighbor carry her groceries, if our long-term motivation is attaining enlightenment so that we can help all beings become free of all their suffering and attain the perfect state of enlightenment as well, then these simple actions bring us closer to enlightenment, and become beneficial for all beings.

Some people immediately feel comfortable with the idea of bodhichitta and can start integrating it into their lives. Others find it more difficult. They may think, "Is there really such a thing as enlightenment?" or "Me becoming enlightened? Helping all beings? I'm not sure... I have trouble just taking care of myself and my family!" For people who feel like this, doing things with bodhichitta can simply mean being as kind as possible, trying to help others and avoid harming them, and learning to be less selfish and more altruistic.

However, it is possible for all of us to develop full-fledged bodhichitta. There are various methods for doing so, which involve meditating on and making our minds familiar with certain thoughts and attitudes. The more our minds become familiar with these, the more bodhichitta will arise naturally and effortlessly.

One method is known as "equalizing and exchanging oneself with others" and involves contemplating five points:

1. Equalizing oneself with others. All beings – I and everyone else – are equal in wanting to be happy and wanting to not suffer. There is no reason why my wish to be happy and free of suffering is more important than anyone else's.

2. The faults of self-cherishing. The self-cherishing attitude (selfishness) – caring more for myself than for others – is the cause of problems, and an obstacle to real peace and happiness. For example:

   - Self-cherishing motivates me to do negative actions such as stealing or saying hurtful words, and thus I create the causes for problems in the future.
   - All the problems I experience in this life are the result of negative karma created in past lives, motivated by selfishness.
   - Self-cherishing causes problems in my relationships, at work, and even when I'm by myself, e.g. feeling lonely, bored, or depressed.

- Self-cherishing hinders my spiritual practice (e.g. I spend a lot of time watching television or going shopping when I could be meditating) and stops me from creating positive karma (e.g. I don't practice generosity as much as I could because I want to keep my money for myself). In these ways, self-cherishing prevents my attainment of happiness in future lives.
- Self-cherishing is one of the biggest obstacles to attaining enlightenment. In fact, it's impossible to become enlightened unless I stop being selfish.

In conclusion, if I wish to be helpful to others in the best possible way, both now and in the future, I must overcome this attitude.

3. The benefits of cherishing others. Unselfishness – cherishing others more than myself – is the cause of all happiness and peace up to enlightenment. This is because:

- Cherishing others motivates me to do positive actions, such as sharing my things with others, helping others when they are in need, etc. The karma I create is the cause of happiness and good experiences in the future.
- The good experiences I have now in my life – being healthy, having enough resources such as food and money, having people who love me, etc. – are the result of positive karma I created in past lives motivated by unselfishness.
- Cherishing others enables me to have more harmonious, satisfying relationships with others in my family, at work, and so on, and thus I have more peace and happiness here and now.
- Cherishing others is the most positive and powerful motivation for spiritual practice. Any actions done with the motivation to help others bring me closer to enlightenment.

4. Exchanging oneself with others. By contemplating the faults of self-cherishing and the benefits of cherishing others, I realize that it's better to be less concerned with myself and more caring towards others. Therefore, I resolve to work on changing my attitude from self-cherishing to cherishing others.

5. Tonglen: giving and taking. This is a powerful meditation for transforming the mind from self-cherishing to cherishing others. Tonglen involves two steps: first, you meditate on compassion, the wish for others to be free from suffering, and then imagine taking their suffering into yourself, using it to annihilate the self-cherishing attitude. Second, you meditate on love, the wish for others to be happy, and imagine giving all your happiness, good qualities, and positive karma to others, making them happy. Chapter 4 of this book contains an explanation of the benefits of tonglen, and there is a meditation on tonglen by Lama Zopa Rinpoche in Chapter 6.

This meditation on equalizing and exchanging oneself with others is the basis of the practice of the five powers, which Rinpoche explains extensively in Chapter 4.

Should we be afraid of death?

In Chapter 1, when discussing the disadvantages of not remembering death, Lama Zopa Rinpoche says that if we do not remember death we will not be afraid of death. And if we do not feel afraid of death we will spend all our time and energy seeking the comfort and pleasures of this life, and will not do any Dharma (spiritual) practice.

Does this mean that it is good to fear death? That we should be afraid of death, as if death is inherently terrifying?

The issue of fear is quite controversial in the West. Many people believe that fear is a negative emotion, something that we should not have if we are spiritual practitioners. They feel that we shouldn't engage in spiritual practice out of fear. And some people think that fear is a sign of weakness, and are ashamed to acknowledge that they have it. Are these ideas and attitudes correct?

Let's leave aside for now the question of whether or not fear is negative. A more fundamental question is: does it exist? Do we have fear – of death or anything else? If we do have fear in our minds or hearts, but we think, "I should not be afraid, fear is negative," or "I should be strong, not afraid," is that helpful? Is that the right way to deal with fear?

Some people have no difficulty recognizing and acknowledging that they are afraid of death, so they are not in denial, but they may have the problem of being so afraid that they avoid the subject of death altogether. That is a problem because they never face their fears and learn how to manage them. Then when death happens, they panic, overwhelmed by fears. We can learn to deal with fear and even overcome it, and as a result we will be able to face death calmly, with acceptance.

There are other people who think they have no fear of death. Some of these people are being honest, but some are in denial. I know, because I used to be like that. When I was in my teens I had a kind of flippant attitude about death, thinking "Oh well, if it happens, it's okay. No problem. I'm not afraid." That attitude changed when I attended my first meditation course in 1974 at Kopan Monastery in Nepal. I had heard teachings on death and the importance of meditating on death, but I did not take them very seriously. One night during the course, there was an earthquake as we sat meditating with Lama Zopa Rinpoche. It was not very strong, but we could hear the voices of people in the nearby villages, crying out in fear, and Rinpoche suddenly said in a serious voice, "Meditate on bodhichitta." My immediate thought was "We're going to die!" and my mind, instead of meditating on bodhichitta, went into total panic. I've never felt such fear in my life, and because we were sitting in meditation (or trying to, anyway) the contents of my mind were especially vivid, like a movie on a big screen. I was frozen with fear, unable to think of anything positive, anything helpful.

After a few moments (which seemed like ages) the earth stopped shaking, the people stopped screaming, everything became calm, and I thought, "Whew! We're not going to die. Thank goodness!" That experience was immensely valuable. I realized how fragile life is, how it can be lost in a moment. I also realized that I was in fact afraid of dying and completely unprepared for death. And I felt certain that when death did happen, I did not want to die in such a state of panic. I wanted to have a peaceful, positive state of mind. So that experience gave me a lot of energy to work on my mind, to learn how to keep it peaceful and positive. Now, when I hear people say "I'm not afraid of death" or "Death is no big deal, we don't need to talk about it or meditate on it," I wonder how well they know their own minds.

We need to check our minds carefully and honestly to see whether or not we are afraid of death. How do you feel when you are almost in a car accident, or when you are watching a scary movie in which someone is being stalked by a killer? What is your reaction when a friend or relative is diagnosed with a terminal illness or when you attend a funeral? In such situations, is your mind completely calm and relaxed or is there tension? Are there knots in your stomach? If there is fear of death in your mind and you deny that fear, you will probably have difficulty later, at the time of death. Instead, you can acknowledge the fear now and learn to deal with it, so that you are better prepared to face death calmly.

How can we deal with fear? A general method is simply to look into the fear and try to understand what it's all about. What exactly are you afraid of? And once you figure that out, check: is there is anything I can do? If there is something that can be done, do it!

For example, you may be afraid of pain. This fear is to some extent unnecessary because not everyone has pain when they die, and for those who do have pain, medication is usually available. If you don't like the idea of medication, you can learn methods such as meditation for dealing with pain. If you are afraid of separating from your loved ones and possessions, you can start to work on overcoming attachment (there are many methods in Buddhism that help you to do that). When I examine my own fear of death,

I find that it's not so much death that I am afraid of, but my reaction to death. I'm afraid of being overwhelmed by disturbing emotions, and unable to stay calm and clear. To counteract that, I am learning how to deal with my mind, how to keep it positive and free of disturbing thoughts.

That is what Lama Zopa Rinpoche is saying. He is saying that if we never think about death and always avoid the subject, we will not recognize our fear of death. And if we don't recognize that fear, we will not do what we need to in order to be free of fear, and then we won't be prepared for death. What we should fear is not death, but dying with an uncontrolled mind, and dying without having done anything positive in our life. And the way to avoid such a death is to train in spiritual practice – Dharma – during our life. It's easy to become so busy with the activities of this life that we don't find the time to do spiritual practice. Therefore, remembering death, especially the fact that it could happen any moment, is a powerful incentive to engage in spiritual practice.

Now let's go back to the question of whether or not fear is negative. It depends on what we are afraid of, if the danger is real or imaginary, and how we deal with our fear. If there is a real danger, and we deal wisely with our fear, it will motivate us to avoid what we are afraid of. For example, fear of being in a car accident motivates us to drive safely. Fear of sickness motivates us to eat well and follow a healthy lifestyle. Fear of the painful consequences of negative actions motivates us to avoid them and to do positive actions instead. Fear of an uncontrolled mind at the time of death motivates us to learn how to keep our minds positive, free of disturbing, negative thoughts. These are constructive ways of working with fears that are realistic. On the other hand, fear can be negative if it is imaginary or exaggerated, or if we do not deal with it wisely but let ourselves be overwhelmed or immobilized.

From a Buddhist perspective, the reason that we have fear is because we have ignorance that sees everything – our self, others, and all things – in an incorrect way. Ignorance is the basis for other delusions such as attachment, wishing never to separate from loved ones and cherished possessions, and aversion, wanting to be distant from unpleasant people and experiences. Any time we examine one of our fears, we will most probably find one or both of these delusions behind it. So from this point of view, we can say that fear is negative and something to be overcome. One of the qualities of a Buddha, an enlightened being, is freedom of all fears. But until we reach the state where we are free from fear, it is best to acknowledge and work wisely with our fears.

Meditation

There are a number of meditations in this book and on the audio MP3 disc that is included with it, and a number of occasions in which Lama Zopa Rinpoche mentions practicing meditation at the time of death. The subject of meditation is vast, far beyond the scope of this book, but a few words here might be helpful to readers who have little experience of it.

In general, the purpose of practicing meditation is to transform the mind from negative to positive. The word for meditation in Tibetan, *gom*, literally means "to be familiar." Meditation involves making our minds familiar with positive attitudes such as love, compassion and wisdom, and de-familiarizing ourselves with negative ones such as anger, attachment and ignorance. By practicing meditation regularly over a period of time, we will have fewer negative thoughts arising in our minds, and more positive ones.

There are many different kinds of meditation, but they can all be included in two categories: placement and analytical. Placement meditation could also be called concentration meditation. It involves focusing the mind on just one object, such as the breath or an image of the Buddha, without thinking about the object or anything else. In order to succeed in this practice we must learn to stop the "chattering" mind, and to cultivate a silent, still, clear state of mind. The purpose of this form of meditation is developing single-pointed concentration, an essential tool for traversing the spiritual path.

Analytical meditation, on the other hand, involves thinking and analyzing. It is used to recognize mistaken concepts and attitudes that we have – those that cause suffering to ourselves and others – and to familiarize ourselves with correct and beneficial ones. The ultimate purpose of this kind of meditation is to develop the wisdom that sees the true nature of things.

The meditations included in this book and audio course are analytical. If you wish to practice them, sit in a place that is as quiet and free of distractions as possible. It's good if you can sit cross-legged, but that's not essential; it's perfectly okay to meditate sitting in a chair. Whichever way you sit, keep your back straight; this enables your mind to be more clear and focused.

Begin the meditation with a few minutes of stilling your mind, letting go of all other thoughts and concerns. Focusing on and counting your breath can help you to do this. Once your mind is calm, generate a positive motivation for doing the meditation, for example, "I wish to practice meditation in order to decrease the negative energy in my mind and to increase my positive qualities such as love, compassion, patience, and wisdom. In this way, I will have more beneficial, positive energy to bring into my interactions with others, and to send out into the world." Or, if you are comfortable with the idea of bodhichitta, you can think, "I am going to do this meditation in order to attain enlightenment so that I can help all beings attain that state as well."

Then begin the actual meditation. If you do not know the points of the meditation from memory, you can have the book open in front of you. Read a portion of the meditation, then close your eyes and contemplate it. Feel free to bring your own ideas and experiences into your contemplation. The point is to generate an actual experience of what you are meditating on. For example, the purpose of doing the nine-point meditation on death is to realize that you are definitely going to die, that it could happen at any moment, and that you must do some spiritual practice in order to be prepared for death and what happens afterwards. These realizations will have a powerful impact on the way you see yourself and your life, and on the way that you live your life.

However, don't expect to have such life-changing experiences right from the beginning of your practice of meditation. It takes time to learn basic skills like sitting still, keeping your mind on the meditation-object instead of wandering away, and dealing with doubts and questions that might come up in your mind during the meditation. Meditation is not easy, and analytical meditation can be particularly tricky. It is ideal if you have access to an experienced meditator who can help you deal with whatever difficulties you encounter in your practice. Otherwise, trying to practice on your own without guidance could result in problems.

At any rate, if you do reach a point in your meditation where you have a strong experience of something such as the need to engage in spiritual practice in preparation for death, then it is best to stop the thinking and analyzing process and focus your mind on that experience as long as possible, even for just a few seconds. When the experience fades, you can return to the analytical process, or conclude the meditation. This method of combining analytical and placement/concentration mediation is how we actually bring about a transformation of our minds.

There is no fixed rule about the length of a meditation session. Initially, you could try meditating for fifteen to twenty minutes, but more or less is also okay. You can experiment with varying lengths of time to see what works best for you, according to your ability and schedule. Lama Yeshe used to say that even five minutes of meditation can be very beneficial. Quality is more important than quantity. A short session in which your mind is very focused, for example, is more worthwhile than a long session where your mind is all over the place.

When it is time to end your meditation session, make a positive conclusion to what you have thought about and experienced. For example, you might resolve to work on particular habits or attitudes which you recognize as potentially disturbing to your mind at the time of death. Finally, remember the motivation you started with and dedicate the positive energy you created during the meditation to that same purpose.

TEACHINGS ON DEATH AND DYING

by Lama Zopa Rinpoche

Meditation is a force to stop problems, not something that you can only practice very quietly somewhere on a mountain. Meditations on death are meant to solve problems; if you don't use them for their intended purpose, what's the point?

chapter 1

Impermanence and Death

Life is so fragile. Its nature is transitory. Life changes after only one year, a month, a week, a day, an hour, a minute, and second by second. There are sixty-five of the shortest instants in the time it takes to snap your fingers, and even in those short split seconds, life is changing.

You might think: "Why should I be surprised that life changes so much? That is natural; let it happen!" To think in this way is very foolish and ignorant, because as life is changing so quickly, in those very short instants we are becoming older. Some may say, "That is natural. I become older; let it happen!" Not caring about becoming old is another wrong attitude. Others want to deny the impermanent nature of their lives; they do not want to see the true nature of it at all. They try to disguise their appearance in the eyes of others, who also play the same game. This is an absolutely vain attempt; such actions are not of the potential knowledge level of the human mind, and their creation is certainly not the purpose of the human rebirth from the Dharma point of view. No artificial effort can change eighty years into sixteen. Age can never decrease in the view of the truly enlightened mind, which fully realizes that the nature of the samsaric body is impermanent, and therefore, in the nature of suffering.

These people's minds have a double illusion: belief in artificial creation (scientific discoveries used to preserve life from ruin and decay) and the wrong conception that a permanent self exists. The first wrong belief causes problems to arise continually. The second wrong idea causes us to become more ignorant, lazy, and careless.

There are two levels of impermanence: 1) gross – changes of matter that happen over long periods of time and 2) subtle – inner changes of mind and invisible changes of matter that happen in the shortest part of a second.

Our minds can't perceive subtle changes of matter; we can see only the gross changes from day to day and hour to hour, such as ruin, death, and so forth. The great meditator Gampopa said: "This vessel-like world that existed at an earlier moment does not do so at a later one. That it seems to continue in the same way is because something else similar arises, like the stream of a waterfall."

Why should we worry about the changes of becoming old? Because as years, months, days, and split seconds are passing and we grow older, the perfect chance of attaining enlightenment given by this human rebirth is ending and I am becoming closer to death. I have the right equipment, a pilot, a spaceship, and enough fuel to make a trip around the universe and visit all the planets. But here I sit, engine running, burning up fuel while my mind is distracted by other things. The longer my mind remains distracted, the more I miss the chance of seeing the planets. As the fuel burns, time grows shorter. However, even this analogy does not adequately show the tragedy of wasting this precious human rebirth.

It is certain that you are not going to live much over one hundred years; you probably won't live past ninety. Even if you are going to live a million years, your life starts to finish at the time of your conception. As soon as your mind enters your mother's womb, your years start running out and the impermanence of your life begins. Even if you are going to live a hundred thousand years, as soon as it begins, your life starts becoming shorter. It changes in the shortest fraction of a second. As even the nanoseconds pass, nothing remains the same; nothing lasts.

As the seconds pass, so do the minutes that are made up by them. As the minutes pass, so do the hours that are made up by them. As the seconds, minutes, and hours pass, life changes. As twenty-four hours pass, so does a day; as thirty days pass, so does a month. As the months pass, so do the years. No matter whether your lifespan is a thousand years or a hundred thousand, you are growing older and decaying – from the time your mind enters your mother's womb.

From the moment life begins, it starts to finish. As each second passes, that much life has finished and you draw closer to death. Similarly, as each minute, hour, day, and month passes, that much of your life is over and you are that much closer to death. Eventually, when a hundred thousand years have passed, the person whose life was that long has reached the time of death.

It has been like this since you were born, since your mind was conceived in your mother's womb. From that time, you have had a certain lifespan. The number of years you have from the time your mind was conceived in your mother's womb until your death is determined by your karma. Your projected lifespan is karmically determined.

Even if your life could be a hundred thousand years, it would still be constantly growing shorter, finishing, becoming closer to death. Therefore, what need is there to mention that our own lives, which are that much shorter, are also finishing? Our lives are so short. Even if our lives are of average span, say sixty or seventy years, from the moment of conception, they become shorter and shorter; they start to finish. As our lives change and decay in the shortest part of a second, that much life has finished and we are that much closer to death.

As many years as you have lived so far, that much of your life has gone; you are that much closer to death and your time to live is that much less. No matter whether you think you are young or old, whatever your age, that much of your life has finished. It is gone forever, irretrievable. And what life you have left is certainly shorter than that which has passed; more years of your life have passed than you have left.

The Advantages of Remembering Death

The Buddhist teachings on death and impermanence are very useful. We should always remember death. If we do, our minds will remain aware of the changes constantly happening within us, of how short the human life is, of how life is becoming shorter every moment. This has great benefit.

Many great yogis started by meditating on the shortness of the human life, impermanence, and death. Their enlightenment, their realizations, and their Dharma practice itself all came from this meditation. Their strength and ability to live an ascetic life in extremely isolated places, to practice the vast and profound subjects and attain the higher paths, to generate the incredible energy required to persevere in their practice - all these things came from thinking about the shortness of the human life, impermanence and death. The fact that they attained enlightenment in that lifetime was also due to this remembrance.

It takes a great deal of energy to reach enlightenment; the quicker you want to receive it, the more energy you will have. If, for example, you want to cover a long distance quickly by car, you need a good machine, good fuel, and the energy to drive. Similarly, it is not easy to attain enlightenment in your lifetime: you need great energy to overcome the difficulties of practicing Dharma and following the path. Where does such energy come from? It comes from remembering the impermanence of life and death. Therefore, this meditation is extremely useful. Even the continual benefit that enlightened beings bring to sentient beings can be traced back to this meditation.

Remembering impermanence and death is also important if you just want to be reborn in the upper realms or free yourself from samsara. Remembering impermanence and death helps put an end to all 84,000 delusions. All the different negative minds - the great root of ignorance, hatred, all the other wrong conceptions, all the obscurations that prevent liberation from samsara and enlightenment - can be terminated by the energy generated through remembering impermanence and death. This meditation is the original cause of the cessation of all these delusions. Therefore, it is very powerful.

If you remember impermanence and death, you can also prevent the arising of temporal negative minds such as greed, ignorance, hatred, pride, jealousy, and so forth – the minds that cause you discomfort, suffering, and confusion. You prevent them from arising because remembering impermanence and death makes you fear death and the shortness of the human life. Therefore, it is very useful in making your mind peaceful, even in the present.

Not only is remembering impermanence and death useful at the beginning of practice – when it persuades you to seek out the Dharma and begin to practice instead of following your negative mind and acting opposite to the Dharma, it is also beneficial during the practice. Once you are on the path, it inspires you to continue your practice. Even though you are following the path, remembering death keeps you from losing your realizations and helps you continue to the higher reaches of the path. It is also useful at the end of your practice.

Finally, at the time of death, this remembrance is useful because it allows you to die peacefully, with happiness, a relaxed mind, and no worries at all. Even though your relatives might be crying and the people around you might be suffering, you can die with great joy, like going on holiday or a picnic. Definitely! The person who has spent his or her life remembering death every day, continuously purifying, creating merit, and creating as little negative karma as possible has no trouble at the time of death.

Is it really possible to be happy at the time of death?

Those who have created great, extensive merit are happy at the time of death. This is definitely possible.

Ordinary people are usually afraid at the time of death, but for the purest Dharma practitioners, death is like returning home or going on a picnic. Intermediate Dharma practitioners are happy and worry-free at the time of death. The lowest Dharma practitioners, at least those who created much merit during their life, aren't upset at the time of death; they are not worried. Because they have done much purification and collected much merit, they are not afraid at the time of death.

Therefore, since there are so many benefits in remembering death, instead of being shocked by all this talk about it, forgetting it, or stopping yourself from remembering it, you should always remember and meditate on the impermanence of life. Why does this topic shock people? Why are people shocked when they are asked their age and the person replies, "Oh, you are so old!"? Because it is opposite to the way they feel, opposite to their wrong conceptions, to what they believe.

People always want to look young, not to age, not to change, but no matter how strong their desire, they have no choice. Therefore, they are shocked when they are told they are old.

No matter how much you don't want it to happen, you can't stop change; you can't stop the natural evolution of the impermanent life. Trying to forget it, not think about it, or disguise it cannot affect the actual evolution.

Artificial change – make up, plastic surgery, and so forth – cannot make you younger, cannot arrest the aging process, cannot prevent decay, cannot stop death. Even if you spend your whole life trying to look young on the outside, you still age and die. You can't stop death by forgetting about it, by never thinking about it, by closing your ears and not listening if somebody else is talking about it. Nothing can stop death, no matter how you try.

Whatever your age, however young-looking you try to remain through external means, the actual evolution is that you are growing older; you are like a piece of rotten fruit painted on the outside to look nice. A painted piece of fruit might look beautiful and fresh, but inside, it decays, loses its taste, shrivels up, and sours. No matter how much it is painted on the outside, nothing stops the actual evolution of decay.

Since we have to go through the natural evolution of life without choice, all these external manipulations don't help. No matter how much we try to disguise what is happening and pretend that it is not, we still have to experience the worries of old age and the suffering of death. Trying to forget these things is not the solution. If someone is coming to kill you, it doesn't help to pretend that it is not happening. Ignoring the fact doesn't avert the danger. You have to do something else.

Therefore, instead of being shocked and trying to escape from the natural way things are, do the opposite – constantly bring impermanence and death to mind. This is much more useful than trying to stop the fear that normally arises from remembering death by ignoring it, and it has so many advantages.

As the great Tibetan yogi Milarepa said, "I fled to the mountains through fear of death, and once there, I realized the absolute true nature of mind. Now, even if death comes to me, I won't be afraid."

This is very tasty, very effective. The great yogi Milarepa's body was something else. Because he spent a long time naked, doing austere practices, leading an ascetic life in the mountains, his body was green, scrawny, and ugly. If he showed up in the West today, he would be arrested; everybody would hate the way he looked. He would be hidden away out of sight.

An austere life is one where you forgo possessions and temporal needs, no matter how difficult it is, bearing whatever hardships arise in order to practice Dharma. Milarepa remembered death and felt afraid, and his fear drove him to the mountains, where he realized the absolute true nature, the reality of the mind, and thus overcame his fear of death. This great achievement originally came from his remembering and fearing the shortness of the human life. We should learn from his example and practice in the same way – remember death and overcome fear of it before it comes. This is the wise approach, wise work, the skillful method; it is much better than what people normally do, which is avoid the fear of death by not thinking about it until it is time to die.

Another Tibetan yogi, who wrote many texts and was in constant communication with the female buddha Tara, also practiced remembering impermanence and death, created much merit, received many realizations, and eventually overcame his fear of death. He said, "When the impermanence of life manifests to me, I won't be afraid. I can be a monk in the morning and take the body of a deity the same afternoon." Not only was he unafraid of death, but he also had the power to take a pure body when he left his ordinary one.

All these benefits that I've mentioned, then, are advantages of re-membering impermanence and death, so this practice is very useful. By remembering death, you stop following your negative mind and therefore create less negative karma. The more you remember death, the better the results you experience. It is very helpful.

The Disadvantages of Not Remembering Death

If you don't remember death, you don't remember Dharma, which is the only method that can fully eliminate the fear of death. How does this work? If you don't remember death, you are not afraid of it. If you are not afraid of death, you become strongly attached to the comfort of this life and you spend most of your time seeking only that comfort. You have one idea after another – to do business, to do this, to do that – all to gain only the comfort of this life. You do one thing, then another, then something else, and this is how your entire life goes, working for attachment, the thought that is attached to the comfort of this life. You don't remember death and because you spend all your time working for this life, you cannot practice Dharma. Then you finish up with great suffering at the time of death – not only have you used your whole life to create the cause of suffering, you also have no happiness or peace of mind when you die.

If you don't remember death, you are controlled by attachment and follow your negative mind, saying: "Oh, I can practice Dharma in a couple of years; there is no hurry. Maybe I'll get to it in a year, in a few months' time." You put it off. Then when the time comes, you again say, "Maybe next month, next year." This is a big danger. Even though you remember Dharma, you postpone your practice in this way. This comes from not remembering impermanence and death strongly or frequently enough.

Another problem is that you might try to practice Dharma, to meditate, but whatever you do doesn't become pure. It is very difficult for your practice to be pure if you don't remember death.

This wrong conception, this intuitive feeling – thinking all the time, every day: "I am going to live for a long time; I am not going to die; I am not going to die today – is the worst hindrance to making your Dharma practice pure. Whatever you are doing – walking, sitting, whatever – the intuitive feeling "I am not going to die today" is always in your mind.

Anybody can say, "Eventually I am going to die; after a long time." This is not enough. Even people who don't meditate think like that. The problem for the meditator and non-meditator alike, especially for those of us who are trying to practice Dharma, is that the wrong conception, "I am not going to die today," means that even though we try to practice Dharma, our practice becomes impure.

How does this thought prevent our practice from becoming pure? Because when we think in this way, we have no fear of death, and because we do not fear death, we always fall under the control of attachment; attachment to the comfort of this life. This is the way it works. Because of the continual feeling "I am not going to die today" we have no fear of death. We are controlled by attachment to the comfort of this life, and therefore, work only for this life. In this way, everything we do becomes the cause of suffering.

Because you aren't afraid of death, even though you try to do something positive, try to meditate, your motivation is not pure; you don't have the strong thought that what you are doing is only for the benefit of future lives. You don't develop complete disregard for this life; you don't have the feeling that the comfort of this life is like used toilet paper, something only to be cast aside. You don't have strong motivation like this.

Even if you do have some idea of future lives, your desire to benefit this life is much stronger. Therefore, even when you try to practice Dharma, the motivation behind your practice is the comfort of this life. Therefore, what you do doesn't become pure

Dharma. If you don't have the strong motivation of wanting to achieve the supreme happiness of enlightenment, the cessation of samsara, or the happiness of future lives, and complete detachment from the comfort of this life, if the intuitive thought "I am not going to die today" constantly arises, your practice becomes impure. Why? Because the pure motivation to do the practice only for those higher goals will not arise.

These disadvantages and advantages are important to know and remember. Otherwise, you will have no interest in meditating on death and impermanence; and you won't have energy for the meditation. If you don't do the meditation, you won't gain all the perfections that come from remembering and meditating on impermanence and death. Therefore, it is very useful to think of the shortcomings and the benefits – what happens if you don't remember these things and what happens if you do. Then you will have the energy to meditate on impermanence and death instead of being shocked by the subject. You will be willing to experience these meditations.

Meditating on Impermanence

When we meditate on the impermanence of this life, it is useful to think like this:

- When you look at a river, think that just as the river flows, life finishes just as quickly.
- As the sun rises and sets, think that life passes just as quickly.
- While you see external things clearly changing – such as incense or candles burning down – you don't see your life finishing in parallel. Pay attention to what is happening around you. Then you will easily be able to understand that your life is finishing without a moment's delay. Just as the oil in a burning lamp is steadily consumed, so too is your life.
- As the seasons pass, so does your life; as summer, autumn, winter, and spring pass quickly by, so does your life, becoming shorter and shorter, finishing more and more quickly.

Relating what you see in the outside world to yourself is extremely useful; it is a type of analytical meditation. It is useful because it prevents your mind from becoming deluded; it makes your mind aware of change, of life becoming shorter, of the brevity of human life, your life.

We see external things going by quickly but never reflect on our own life. We are always planning on having a long life; we completely believe that we will continue to exist for a long time. We are totally unaware of the way in which our life is actually evolving: finishing quickly every moment. The same evolutionary changes we see outside of ourselves are happening within; this is the actual evolution, but we don't recognize it.

Not realizing how quickly and relentlessly life is finishing becomes the greatest hindrance to making our whole life pure, to living in a positive way, to spending our entire life in the Dharma. Because we have the wrong conception that we are not going to die soon and instead are going to live a long time, we don't remember death, don't think of Dharma, and don't make any arrangements for our next life. Since we don't think about death and how short life is, we have no fear. Because we have no fear of the brevity of life, death, and the suffering that follows, we don't change our lives. Even though we might know all about meditation or be great Dharma scholars, if we remain unaware of the actual evolution of life, if we have no wisdom, we won't change our lives; we won't make them pure.

Being worried and afraid at the time of death doesn't help because at that point there is nothing we can do. No matter how great our suffering, fear, and worry knowing we are now going to die, there is nothing we can do. Whatever negative karma we have created, whatever the huge amount of garbage in our minds, we have to carry it all. Since we have created the cause, we have to suffer each result. Then, no matter how much incredible fear and worry we have, it doesn't help at all because there is no time to practice. Our time is up, finished, gone. There is nothing we can do to solve this problem.

If your house is susceptible to damage by flood, it is wise to check beforehand how great the danger is. If you find the danger is real, you feel afraid. Because of that fear, you dam the river or make other arrangements to protect your house, family, and property from being ruined by floodwaters. When you know you are safe, your life becomes peaceful; you have no worries. In the same way, it is necessary to make arrangements to protect your peace of mind before the flood of death arrives. Before death arrives, research the danger and act accordingly.

If you don't fear danger, you'll never make the necessary arrangements to protect yourself. Therefore, you have to meditate on impermanence and death in order to realize the danger, feel afraid and do what's necessary to protect yourself.

meditation

Life is Finishing Quickly

Think how a lifespan of 100,000 years finishes, by seconds, months, and years. Every second, month, and year, a life of 100,000 years becomes shorter and shorter. 100,000 years is made up of a certain number of seconds, a certain number of fractions of a second, which start running out from the moment of conception in the mothers' womb. As soon as life begins, as each split second passes, the whole collection of split seconds starts to finish; the entire collection of split seconds that equal 100,000 years runs out split second by split second. Each moment, the life of 100,000 years becomes shorter. In this way, by subtracting each split second from the whole, the total number becomes less and life finishes. Life finishes so quickly.

Think, "Since I was conceived in my mother's womb, since my mind entered the fertilized egg, my karmically determined lifespan – sixty, seventy years – has been decreasing. My projected lifespan has a finite number of hours, minutes, and seconds, and within that time, there is a finite number of split seconds. As each split second passes, each second becomes shorter and finishes. As each second passes, each minute becomes shorter and finishes. As each minute passes, each hour becomes shorter and finishes. As each hour passes, each day becomes shorter and finishes. As each day passes, each week becomes shorter and finishes. As each week passes, each month becomes shorter and finishes. As each month passes, each year becomes shorter and finishes. And as each year passes, I have one year less to live.

"If I am going to live to the age of seventy, as each year passes – each year that is made up of split seconds, seconds, minutes, hours, days, weeks, and months – my life is finishing. As many split seconds as there are in my karmic lifespan, as each one passes, my life is becoming closer to its end, continuously finishing. From the time of my conception, from the time my mind entered my mother's womb, my life has been becoming shorter and shorter, without pause. From that moment, my seventy years have been running out. My life is like a pile of rice, from which grains are removed one by one. As each grain is removed, the pile gradually runs out. In just this way, as each moment passes, my life is finishing and I am becoming older and closer to death.

"As each second that makes up my seventy years passes, I am becoming closer to death. Day and night, whatever I am doing – eating, drinking, sleeping, talking, meditating – moment by moment, all the time, I am becoming closer to death. From the time of my conception up until now, a certain number of seconds of my life has passed; a certain number of days, months, and years have passed. Since that time, I have been running towards death without even a split second's pause.

"If I am going to live seventy years, within that time I have a certain number of breaths. There is a fixed number; it is not infinite. Therefore, each time I breathe, my life is finishing. As the total number of breaths that makes up my life decreases, I am becoming closer to death. In one day, I have a certain number of breaths, several thousand, and as each one finishes, I am becoming closer to death, just like an animal being led to slaughter.

"As a goat is led from its pen to where it will be butchered, each step brings it closer to being killed, closer to death. The goat doesn't know that with each step, it is becoming closer to death. I am just like that pitiful, ignorant animal; with each breath, with the passing of each split second, I remain unaware that I am becoming closer to death.

"My life is becoming closer to death just as a stone thrown into the air continuously becomes closer to hitting the ground without a moment's delay. Just like that my life is constantly becoming closer to death. No matter how much I say that I am alive, every moment I am becoming closer to not being alive, closer to my death."

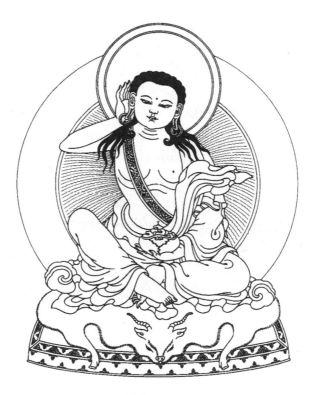

Milarepa

Meditators who have real, true, deep understanding and experience of impermanence and death are never shocked when they hear "renounce this life." Such words only please their minds. Those who realize impermanence and death are only too happy to practice that which is most powerful to stop delusions.

chapter 2

The Nine-Point Meditation on Death

Why am I talking about death? Perhaps you think, "My country is full of danger; people are always dying. I've heard it all before. What's the point of hearing it again?" But this is different. Actually, if we looked the right way at all the examples of impermanence around us, it would be easy to understand by ourselves, but we don't do this. No matter how many outer examples of impermanence we see, we don't realize impermanence on our own.

Even animals are afraid of death – when they are threatened, when they fall – but that is useless. We often feel afraid of death – when we are in an accident, when we are sick – but these feelings don't last. After a day or two, when the danger has passed, we no longer feel afraid and what happened becomes useless because we didn't use it to practice Dharma.

Therefore, it is not enough to bring up a feeling of fear of death for just a couple of minutes; that is not the point. It is necessary to make the fear of death last for more than a few minutes, more than an hour. Why? Because you can't complete the practice of Dharma in an hour. You have to make the feeling last until you know you can be reborn according to your choice, or at least until you are fully confident of having achieved the lowest purpose of this meditation, which is not suffering at the time of death. It is necessary to make this feeling last in order to receive the higher, more difficult realizations; that is the purpose of meditating on impermanence and death.

Even ordinary people who know nothing about Dharma sometimes think, "I will die in a while, after a long time." But if you have the actual realization, if you really fear death, if you have had the experience of impermanence through meditation, then you can never fall asleep while meditating, for example. Sometimes you might meditate for a couple of minutes and then your mind will go off on a picnic. If you have understood and realized impermanence, your mind will be so strong that this sort of thing will never happen; your mind will never be easily distracted. Things like falling asleep during meditation, being easily distracted, and finding it difficult to focus on the subject show that you need energy, that you need to work on a better understanding of impermanence and death. If you haven't experienced impermanence through meditation, if you don't have this realization, then any little problem will disturb your meditation.

Meditators who have real, true, deep understanding and experience of impermanence and death are never shocked when they hear "renounce this life." Such words only please their minds. Those who realize impermanence and death are only too happy to practice that which is most powerful and beneficial to stop delusions, no matter how difficult. For such people it is not difficult. Why are we not capable of this? It is because we haven't realized the impermanence of life and death.

Since meditation is meant to stop your problems, you need to know how to do it, so practicing for just a day or two is not enough to learn; hearing someone explain something once and then just working on that is also not enough.

The Nine-Point Meditation on Death

The Tibetan Buddhist tradition contains an extremely effective meditation on death called the Nine-Point Meditation on Death. It is presented with three roots, nine reasons, and three conclusions:

1. Death is definite.
    • No being has ever escaped death.
    • I am constantly becoming closer to death.
    • There is not much time to practice Dharma.

Conclusion: I must practice Dharma.

2. The time of death is indefinite.
   - The lifespan of human beings is not fixed.
   - More conditions endanger life than support it.
   - This body is extremely fragile.

Conclusion: I must practice Dharma immediately.

3. Nothing can help at the time of death except my Dharma practice.
   - Wealth can't help.
   - Friends and relatives can't help.
   - Your body can't help.

Conclusion: I must practice Dharma purely.

Death is Definite

Death is inevitable because no being has ever existed in the realms of samsara without continuously suffering death and rebirth. At this moment, if I really check up within myself, I can find neither evidence nor guarantee that my life will continue for any definite period.

Think from the depths of your mind, "After some time, this whole world will become completely empty. I will also cease to exist on this earth." Feel the complete emptiness of all these things and conclude, "Therefore, death is definite."

Think, "There is no cooperative cause or condition that can stop death; there is no external condition that can stop death. As it has not been possible to prevent death from the time the world began until now, death is definite. Also, the lifespan cannot be made longer and spontaneously decreases, therefore, death is certain to occur." Bring to mind your own life when thinking these thoughts.

"Also, my death will occur before I have had much time to spend practicing Dharma. Nothing external can prevent it and when the time comes for me to die, even the best hospitals and the latest medicines cannot help. No matter where I go, I can't escape it.

"If I think back to my parents, my parents' parents, their parents, and on and on back through my ancestors, there are so many, an infinite number. Now not one of them exists. All those previous generations have gone; not one of them remains." Think of your parents, your grandparents, your great-grandparents who have died. "Therefore, it is certain that I will also die. Just as they have ceased to exist, so will I. Soon it will be my turn to die. Therefore, my death is definite."

The Time of Death is Indefinite

Generally speaking, the lifespan of the beings in this world is not definite. It is not fixed at a hundred years or a thousand years as it is in some other realms. In this world, the lifespan varies. Therefore, the time of death is uncertain, not definite. For example:

- People come to the East from the West but there is no certainty that they will return. Before it is time to return, they die. The time of death is uncertain in this way.
- Even though they might have returned to the West, they die before returning home.
- Many people go to sleep but die before they awaken.
- Many people start a meal but die before they finish.
- Many people go out by car but die before returning home.
- Many people are born but die before reaching adulthood.
- Many people are conceived but die before they are born
- Many people go out to play sports but die before the game is over.
- Many people buy new clothes but die before they have time to wear them.
- Many people start to read a book but die before they finish.
- Many people plan a project but die before they can complete it.

- Many people go to war but die before they return home.
- Many people go to work but die before they collect their salary.
- Many people start to talk but die before completing what they wanted to say.
- Many people breathe out but die before they can breathe in.

These are just a few examples of how the actual time of death is uncertain. Just as you see these things happening around you, it is necessary for you to put those examples on yourself, to meditate that what is happening to others can happen to you. It is important to think, "One day I will also die somehow, before I have time to complete what I am doing." Just as you see others dying before they have time to finish what they are doing, you have to see the same thing happening to you. This is a very effective way to meditate. It is certain that you are going to die either during the day or night, in the morning or the afternoon, without finishing something. You breathe out but die before you can breathe back in. It is certain to happen to you, that you will die somehow or other, according to your karma, either at home or while you are out.

You also have to think how temporal needs can become the cause of death; how there are more conditions that endanger life than support it. Therefore, the time of death is uncertain.

Even things that support life can endanger life; food, for example. People die while eating meat or fish, when a bone becomes stuck in their throat. Others die when a house collapses on them. Some are killed by others in arguments over money or in drunken brawls. Others overdose on drugs. Even things that are supposed to support life can destroy it. Therefore, the actual time of death is indefinite.

And this body is extremely fragile, like a water bubble. Even a slight movement can cause injury. Therefore, it is so easy to endanger this life. For this reason, too, the time of death is indefinite.

The time of death is uncertain because it occurs when life ends according to previous karma, when factors sustaining life are unavailable, and through ignorance.

Check in your own mind whether or not you can perceive when you will die. Also check if it is sure to happen only after a long time, after ten years; see if you can be sure of living that long or not. Also check to see if you can be sure of still being alive tomorrow, as you tend to think. You tend to think that you will live for a long time; is it definite that you will live until tomorrow? What reasons do you have for thinking that you will still be alive then? Similarly, check up if you can be sure of being alive tonight, if you will live long enough to go to bed. What proof do you have that you will live that long? If you can't find any proof that you will definitely exist that long, then you can't be sure of being alive long enough to go to bed.

Perhaps you think: "I have this intuitive feeling that I will exist. I don't see anything to indicate that I will die at such and such a time; I just have this instinctive feeling." You talk a lot about your instincts, but this instinctive feeling that you are going to continue to exist will carry on until you die. Even if you were going to die a minute from now, you would still have that feeling. That instinctive feeling is the greatest hindrance to Dharma practice.

Many people worry, thinking, "What is the method to stop distractions? I can't concentrate. I can't do this, I can't do that." Why do they have these problems? It is because they are distracted by the instinctive thought that feels, "I will not die now; I will exist. I won't die now; I won't die today." This instinctive feeling that we always have creates hindrances that prevent our concentration from lasting. This disturbing conception should be stopped by meditation on impermanence and death.

Imagine a person walking through a tiger-infested forest. He is constantly aware of the danger of being attacked by a tiger, so he is always on the alert. He doesn't dare spend even a few minutes gazing at something without watching for tigers. Why does he spontaneously watch for tigers? It is the same with somebody who realizes that the time of death is indefinite, who always feels death might come today, in an hour or a minute, who always thinks the opposite of the way we think. We always think, "I am not dying. I won't die now," but the person who has realized the indefinite time of death is the complete opposite. The meditator thinks, "I will definitely die in an hour, at this time, tonight." This is completely opposite to our usual idea. Because the person thinks, "I will die now, in a minute, in an hour," he or she has incredibly great energy to make every action perfect and pure. Therefore, if you meditate with this thought, you won't have any hindrances to meditation; your mind won't be easily distracted. Your concentration will last much longer because this thought and the fear that comes with it does not allow you to fall under the control of hindrances.

The Death of the Buddha

When Guru Shakyamuni Buddha passed away, he took off his robes, lay down, and said to his disciples, "This is the tathagata's last holy body, so you must look at it." A tathagata is an arya being who has gone beyond all suffering and illusory mind, so when he said "tathagata," he meant himself. Then he gave his last teaching: "All causative phenomena are impermanent. This is the last teaching of the tathagata." Then he passed away.

This was his last teaching; this was his bequest to us sentient beings. This was the most important thing he had to leave us – a teaching on impermanence. Then he passed away. When he asked his disciples to look at the last holy body of the tathagata, many of them fainted and some arhats even passed away themselves; they couldn't bear his passing.

The very last thing he left, his very last teaching – like a will that ordinary people leave that talks about money or whatever it is that the dying person is most hung up on, the most precious thing to the dying person – the most beneficial thing that Guru Shakyamuni Buddha could leave, the most important thing for us to realize and understand was impermanence. Therefore, he ended his life with a teaching on impermanence; his entire teaching ended with this. This is what he told us: "You sentient beings should practice Dharma; if you don't, there is impermanence and death."

In saying that, he meant suffering. This one word, impermanence, shows the entire range of samsaric suffering: "You sentient beings should practice Dharma because you are living in suffering, living in impermanence, under the control of death."

When you are meditating on death, another useful technique is to remember and count up all your relatives and friends who have died. Earlier, we meditated mainly on the generations of ancestors who had passed away, but here I am talking about those you met in this life.

Many of my own relatives and friends of this life have passed away – lay people, monks, lamas and many other friends. I never knew my grandfather, even as a small child. I remember only my grandmother – gray hair, rosary, always sitting by the kitchen fire. During the time I was away in Tibet, she was sick and later went blind. My uncle looked after her for many years, giving her food, taking her out to the bathroom, bringing her back in. He offered service to his mother for a long time, and in between taking care of her, he did prostrations. During that time, while he was taking care of his mother, she died.

Then there is my father. About the time I was due to come out of my mother's womb he had already gone to his next rebirth. When I was very small, all of us children would sleep together at night under our father's long-sleeved coat – his *chuba*, as it is called in Tibetan. It was made of animal hide with fur inside. We all slept under our dead father's coat, and sometimes we would say, "This belonged to Dad."

My mother had several other children, but many of them died before I was born. Now there are just three of us left. Soon all these will also be gone and only their names will remain, with people saying, "Such-and-such a person did this," where nobody can see their physical body any longer.

Then there is the first Western pen friend I had, when I was in India. Our schoolteacher was a Buddhist nun; I think she must have been one of the first Western nuns. Originally she was Christian, then later she traveled around Ceylon, where she took precepts from a Theravadan guru, and then she went to India, where and lived and worked. Around this time, the Tibetan uprising of 1959 occurred and many Tibetans escaped to India. This nun was amongst those sent by the relief committee of the Indian government to look after the Tibetan refugees. Where she worked, the refugees were mainly monks from Lhasa.

One of the ways in which she helped the monks was by finding them pen friends in the West with whom they could correspond. The pen friend she found for me was a Jewish lady living in London. Sometimes she would send me photos of herself, some when she was young and some as she was at the time, which was very old. I was confused because I was quite young and didn't know which one was her. I didn't realize that they were pictures of the same person; I thought they were two different people.

People recognized her as having a good personality and being wise. I think she also wrote books, although I didn't read any of them. She wrote me letters for seven years; each week, so many letters. My room was full of her letters. I replied only occasionally; maybe only three or four times altogether. She was more than eighty-seven, but at that time there wasn't much I could do to help her. She really wanted to understand Dharma, but I couldn't communicate much in English myself, and there weren't any other Tibetans at that place who could write well in English either.

Then her flood of letters stopped and I wondered what had happened. I think she thought that if she told me that she was going into hospital for an operation, I would worry; that is why she didn't write. When she got out of hospital she tried to write but her handwriting was no good; she didn't have the energy to form the letters properly. She couldn't even finish the letter she was writing and had some girl help her complete it. That was the last one I got, where she said she had just been released from hospital.

After that, I had a dream that I was near my house and someone handed me a white letter. The next day, I received a letter exactly like that from her friend, who was the pen friend of another lama, explaining that she had died. Then the more than one thousand monks who lived there did pujas for her; also His Holiness's gurus and other high lamas prayed for her to find a better rebirth. Around that time I'd sent her a gift, but I'm not sure she received it. She was cremated and her ashes were scattered outside in her garden. She gave the paintings I had sent her from India to a local Tibetan center before her death. This is just a little story of impermanence.

Just as this happens to other people, the same thing will happen to us. Our first Western student, the nun Zina, was planning to come to Kathmandu and Dharamsala to receive teachings from our gurus; she made many plans to do all these precious things. However, just before it was time for her to come down from the mountains where she was in retreat, she suddenly got sick. Three or four days later, she was dead. While she was ill for those few days, she lay down in bed, but just before she died, she sat up, holding her rosary in her hand. Her daughter was there, looking her in the face and crying, "Please, mother, don't die." The day she died her daughter cried a lot, but a couple of days later she was back to normal, playing in the yard.

Even though Zina was sick, she had a little time to prepare for death. She was fully expecting to do all the things she planned, but all of a sudden her life finished, before she had time to do them. Still, she was very lucky she could die as a nun – luckier than people who die in America in their beautiful, expensive apartments surrounded by all their relatives and possessions. She died in a very simple, tiny room, having spent most of the previous year in retreat. Also, she had the constant wish to help other people, especially Westerners, but was always worried that she was incapable of doing so. She wasn't even able to sign the last letter she sent us.

At the Time of Death, Only My Dharma Practice Can Help
Buddha Shakyamuni said:

> It is unsure whether tomorrow or the next life will come first. Therefore, it is more worthwhile and wise to be prepared for the future life than for tomorrow.

This is very logical. Even after an hour, you are more likely to be dead than alive. Why is it more certain that you will be dead? Since death is definite, it is certain that you will not exist permanently; therefore, death is more certain than continued existence, even at this time. Thinking like this is very, very useful.

If you check up with your own mind, you will see that this is not true just because Guru Shakyamuni Buddha said so; it is the factual evolution. Because death is more definite than continued existence, even at this time, it is more profitable for you to do something that benefits your future lives than to do something for this body alone. You can never be sure when you will have to leave this body, when you will no longer have it. Thinking like this is especially useful when you become angry, for example. At such times it is more helpful to think about death than the profound teachings on emptiness, which is something that you don't really understand. Generally speaking, thinking about emptiness is profound, but when you are experiencing an immediate problem, thinking about death is even more profound.

When you are having a mental problem with somebody – extreme greed, attachment to possessions or a person, anger, pride, or any other negative mind states – in order to stop creating negative karma and make your mind peaceful, to release confusion, try to think, "Guru Shakyamuni Buddha said that death is more likely than continued existence, so if I'm going to die right now, if my breath is going to stop right away, what's the use of being angry? Why be angry, proud, or attached?" There is no use whatsoever. You can't take the person to whom you are attached into your future life. It is completely useless. All you are doing is creating the cause of suffering. Thinking like this is very useful. Whenever attachment to other people arises, think, "It is more definite that I will leave this body than remain in it. There is no guarantee that I won't leave my body right now." Think in the depths of your mind that you are about to leave your body.

If you do this properly, all of a sudden, the uncomfortable feeling, the negative mind will subside, or relax. You will see no purpose in becoming angry; you will discover by yourself that it is meaningless. In this way, you won't cause problems for others and your mind will relax; you will stop creating negative karma and confusion. This is really practical; this is using meditation in the actual critical time. This is real, practical meditation. Meditation is a force to stop problems, not something that you can only practice very quietly somewhere on a mountain. Meditations like these on death are meant to solve problems; if you don't use them for their intended purpose, what's the point?

Do people or material possessions help to ease or prevent death?
At the hour of death, even the entire Pacific Ocean filled with numberless jewels cannot prevent death from occurring. Neither people – relatives, friends, or others – nor any amount of personal strength or fame can prevent death. Instead of helping, these things only contribute to greater suffering.

How do my attachments cause great suffering at death?
At the time of death, we realize that we are separating from our possessions and loved ones, and tremendously strong attachment and fear arise. Our worry is far greater than usual worry, such as that arising from the separation of a couple or from parents. The physical body creates much suffering and, although we have cared more for it than for any other being's body, it now becomes like our own enemy.

At the hour of death, the king and the beggar are exactly equal in that no amount of relatives or possessions can affect or prevent death. But who is the richer at the time of death? If the beggar has created more merit, then although he looks materially poor he is really the rich man. From the Dharma point of view, the mind that has prepared itself for the journey into the next life has the real riches.

If material possessions and relatives and friends are so meaningless and ineffectual at the time of death and cause suffering, becoming enemies, why do we attach so much importance to them and spend so much time caring for them?

We have been attached to the physical body, providing it with all life's comforts, yet still this care has not ended, and it continues to cause us problems. Has this care really any end? Wouldn't it be better to spend life working for something that can be finished?

Why is your body described as an enemy? Because as you feel that you are going to separate from it, you become extremely anxious; you don't want to leave it. Instead of helping you solve your problem at that time, strong attachment to your body only causes you to remain longer in samsara, to always be trapped in the circle of the bondage of suffering, rebirth, and death. And the same trouble and worry you have with your body - attachment, fear of leaving it, not wanting to do so - you have with your possessions and relatives; you feel very upset at having to leave them. Padmasambhava said:

> The vision of this life is like last night's dream. All meaningless actions are like ripples on a lake.

The dream you had last night was so short; from beginning to end, it was over so quickly. In a dream you might feel as if you have been on a long journey or spent many years doing something, but actually, a dream is just a few minutes in duration. Whatever good things happen in a dream are over quickly. This is one reason why Padmasambhava likens life to a dream - they both finish so quickly. Life is over so soon, like a dream.

No matter what you enjoy in a dream, when you awaken, it is all gone. You might dream that you were successful in business; you made billions of dollars and you feel so happy, but when you wake up, not a single dollar remains. Everything you do in a dream is of no use. In exactly the same way, no matter what you do in this life - how much money you make, how many possessions you accumulate, how successful your business, how happy you are - it is all like last night's dream. Not a single atom of it can be carried into your next life. Just as what you do in a dream is meaningless, so too are all the things you do for just this life.

Ripples on a lake comes and go. Things done for only this life are like that; such actions are endless. No matter how much you work, it can never finish. This quotation from the great yogi Padmasambhava is very powerful.

By caring only for my physical body, I am like a person who will die tomorrow anyway, but goes to the hospital today for expensive treatment. Any temporal happiness is meaningless and only results in suffering, never helping to end the cycle of death and rebirth. At the time of death, numberless relatives, every possession – even numberless universes full of numberless jewels – and my body, which I have cared for more than any other, must all be left behind. They are of as little use as a single hair. At death, neither can be taken with the mind; in effect, there is no difference between all the world's possessions and one tiny hair.

This is also very helpful to think about when you are meditating on death. If you reflect on the fact that you are more certain to die now than to keep on living, and that neither your body nor any of your possessions can be carried with you, that at the time of death these things are useless as a single hair, you will see how meaningless they really are. When you see that all your possessions and a single body hair are equal in value, you will come to see your possessions – which you think are so terribly important – as no longer important.

When meditating on the above topics, see which parts are more effective for your mind, and focus on those. In general, it is good to remember all of them, but if you find certain parts more difficult, focus on the parts that are more effective for you and then amplify them according to your own wisdom and experience in order to see things more clearly.

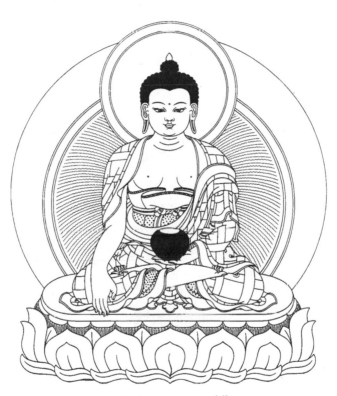

Shakyamuni Buddha

At this point in the death process, the yogis - those meditators who have spent their lifetimes in meditation and practiced various tantric methods, who have observed karma well and kept their precepts purely - use the methods they have been practicing all their lives. This is the moment they have been waiting for.

chapter 3

The Process of Dying

At the time of death, the elements that make up our physical bodies– earth, water, wind, and fire – are absorbed into each other, one after the other. Because of this, many changes appear to the dying person as feelings and visions. At the time of death, the mind separates from the body. The final moment of death comes when the most subtle mind splits from the body, and this also is accompanied by physical signs.

At death, the person who has created much non-virtuous karma suffers disturbing hallucinations that are the result of his past negative actions. A very frightening physical situation occurs because of these fearsome visions. A person who has created virtuous karma experiences a peaceful death. A person dying with an indifferent mind, neither virtuous or non-virtuous, experiences neither pleasure nor suffering.

The process of a natural death – i.e., a death which is not sudden or traumatic – proceeds like this: First, the aggregate of form is absorbed. At the same time, the great mirror wisdom – our ability to clearly see many objects at the same time, as a mirror reflects many objects together – also absorbs. The earth element absorbs, and the physical body becomes very thin and loses power, the hands and legs become very loose, and we feel very uncontrolled, as if being buried under a great weight of earth. Our eye sense base is absorbed, and it becomes impossible to control or move our eyes. Finally, the "inner subtle form" is absorbed. The color of the physical body fades and the body loses its strength completely. Internally, we see a trembling silver-blue mirage, like water in the heat.

Next, the aggregate of feeling is absorbed. Our bodies no longer experience physical pleasure, pain, or indifference. At the same time, the wisdom of equality, which sees all feelings of happiness, suffering and indifference as having the same nature, is absorbed. We no longer remember those feelings perceived with the sense of mind as distinct from those perceived by the physical body. The water element is absorbed, and all the liquids of the body – urine, blood, saliva, sperm, sweat, etc. – dry up. The ear sense base is absorbed and we can no longer hear. The inner sound is absorbed, and we no longer hear even the customary buzzing in the ears. Internally, we experience a vision of smoke, like the room is filled with incense.

Next, the aggregate of perception is absorbed. We no longer recognize our relatives and friends or know their names. Along with that, the wisdom of discriminating awareness is absorbed, and the fire element is absorbed. The heat of the physical body disappears and the capacity to digest food ceases. The nose sense base is absorbed and inhaling becomes difficult and weaker, while exhaling becomes stronger and longer. The inner sense of smell is absorbed and our noses no longer detects smells. Internally, we experience a vision of sparks of fire, trembling like starlight.

Then the aggregate of compounded phenomena is absorbed. Our bodies can no longer move. At the same time, the all-accomplishing wisdom is absorbed. This is the wisdom of attainment that remembers outer work and success and their necessity. We lose the idea of the necessity and purpose of outer work. The air element absorbs and our breathing ceases. The taste sense base is also absorbed, and the tongue contracts and thickens and its root turns blue. The tactile organ is absorbed, and we no longer perceive soft nor rough sensations. The inner taste sense is absorbed, and we can no longer detect the six different tastes. Internally, we experience a vision of a dim red-blue light, like the last flickering of a candle.

Finally, the aggregate of consciousness is absorbed. This consists of the eighty gross superstitions and their foundations, motion.

"Superstitions" means the gross illusive mind, the dualistic, wrong-conception mind. At this point, we have the following visions. First we see the white vision, which is like a very clear sky, like that in autumn, full of the brightness of the moon. Then we experience the red vision, which is like a copper-red reflection in the sky. Then we experience the dark vision which is a vision of empty darkness, like a dark and empty space. Lastly, we experience the clear light vision. This is a vision of complete emptiness, very clear, like the sky of an autumn dawn. This is the vision of the final death. At this time, the time of actual death, the gross mind – that which holds gross objects – ceases, but only momentarily. Due to karma, the seed of it is always there. Now the mind has completely separated from the body. It is possible that ordinary people stay in this stage for some time, but don't recognize it. Highly realized yogis are able to recognize all the visions of the death process, and can stay in this stage, meditating in the void for months.

As you can see, different visions come and go: mirage, smoke, sparks, flame. Then the white vision, like an autumn moon rising or snow on the ground; then red; then dark, like the complete darkness of a dark room, like you are suddenly falling into darkness.

After the dark vision comes the clear light vision, emptiness. But this is not *shunyata*; not that emptiness. If it were, it would be an effortless realization, achieved without meditation. It is not shunyata, but an emptiness like that of the sky at dawn, devoid of the white, red, and dark visions.

Generally, it is not permitted to give the details of these methods openly. However, at this point in the death process, the yogis – those meditators who have spent their lifetimes in meditation and practiced various tantric methods, who have observed karma well and kept their precepts purely – use the methods they have been practicing all their lives. This is the moment they have been waiting for. They can remain in meditation in the clear light for many days or even weeks. The duration varies; it depends upon the meditator.

During that time, there is no smell of decay. They smell the same as when they were alive. Also, they look very magnificent, totally different from an ordinary person dying. Ordinary people – those who didn't practice Dharma during their life, who didn't observe karma well, or who created many negative actions – appear very afraid when they die. Their eyes get wide and they cry because they have many fearful visions. They thrash their limbs about, move their hands as if they are trying to grab hold of something, and might become incontinent. Many things happen like this.

Many Tibetan lamas have passed away in meditation since coming to India. Ordinary Indian people never believed that such things as passing away while sitting in meditation were possible because they never saw it happen. Their usual concept was that the moment a person died, he or she should be taken out and burnt. Otherwise, the body would start to smell. Many Tibetan monks in India had to go to the hospital and, if they died there, it was difficult to receive permission to leave them alone for a while because the doctors would never listen. They would want the body taken out immediately. Their concept was that as soon as the breath stops, the person is dead. Therefore, Indians who saw high lamas in meditation after death were very surprised. Far from there being a bad smell in the room, there was a fantastic sweet smell due to the power of their realizations.

These visions, including the clear light vision, also occur between sleeping and dreaming, and between dreaming and awakening, but they pass very quickly. The great meditators first practice here. Once they can control their dreams, they know for sure that they will be able to employ these profound methods during their actual death. Thus, you can see from your own inability to do this during sleep how impossible it will be for you to be conscious enough to practice these methods during death, to be conscious enough to recognize the visions as they evolve during the death process.

All these visions, including the clear light, are ordinary occurrences that all beings experience, unless their death is sudden, as in an accident, murder and so forth. Even ordinary people experience the gradual absorption of the eighty gross superstitions after the breathing stops, before the white, red, and dark visions occur.

The dark vision occurs when the very subtle mind is enclosed in the seed at the heart. This seed, like a tiny bean, is composed of two hemispheres, like a couple of lids put together. The moment of death occurs when this seed opens and the very subtle mind leaves the body. The sign that this has happened is that a trickle of red blood comes out of the person's nose and a white fluid exudes from the sex organ. It usually takes up to three days for all this to happen, although with certain diseases, these fluids don't come out. When the great meditators have completed their meditation, the red and white fluids come out.

The Intermediate State (Bardo)

Until cognition becomes unclear and powerless, the mind retains its habitual attachment to the self. Because of this attachment, as the cognition weakens, the wrong concept arises that "I am becoming non-existent." This causes fear of losing the I. These thoughts create attachment to and craving for the body, which in turn leads to birth in the intermediate state, the state between the death of this life and the birth of the next life.

As the person enters the intermediate state, the visions that occurred during the death process re-occur but in the reverse order: dark, red and white. Then the eighty superstitions arise.

The intermediate state body is indestructible, like a vajra; like diamond. It has no resistance; nothing can resist it. It also has certain karmically derived psychic powers. It can instantly arrive wherever it thinks of being. But it also undergoes much suffering, for example, feeling as if it is buried under ground and being pressed down by huge mountains. It also has illusory visions, but not realizing that these are projected by its own mind, it becomes very frightened. It feels as if it is being blown about uncontrollably from place to place by a strong red wind or a fierce storm, or caught in a noisy fire, or drowning in an ocean with huge, wrathful waves. It might see karmically created yamas - monsters with terrifying bodies and fearful animal heads - chasing it, shouting, trying to beat and destroy it. It has many frightening experiences like these. There is no time to relax in the intermediate state; there is so much fear and suffering.

If the intermediate state being could recognize its previous life's body, it would be able to re-enter it, but it can't. Once the consciousness leaves, it completely forgets its past life.

The life of each intermediate state body is seven days. Sometimes it will find rebirth before the first seven days are up, in which case it dies and goes through the evolutionary death process again, very quickly, and finds itself in its next life's body. If this doesn't happen after seven days, the intermediate state body dies and it takes another similar one. This process can happen up to a maximum of seven times, forty-nine days. The intermediate state cannot last longer than that. Therefore, Tibetans do pujas for the deceased every seven days after death for seven weeks, the last one being on the forty-ninth day.

Describing the death process another way, we can say that when we die, it is like we have fallen asleep, dreaming is like being in the intermediate state, and waking from a dream is like being reborn.

The most important practice is bodhichitta, then the five powers. Learn these things and put them into practice. You should remember the five powers every day and be ready to die on any day, because it can happen at any time. This is my advice to you regarding the fear of death.

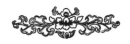

chapter 4

Preparing for Death

Dealing with the Fear of Death

Prepare the mind every day in life. Practice the five powers so that you can apply them at the time of death (*Chapter 5 discusses the five powers in detail*). If you can practice this, you won't need to practice *phowa* and so forth, since the practice of the five powers becomes phowa. Even if you practice phowa, what will make it successful is the basis of having integrated the five powers into your daily life and practiced them as you near the death time. Then, even if you do not die, you will still have created so much merit.

Dying with Bodhichitta

The main thing is to practice bodhichitta. Dying with bodhichitta is the best way to die, as you've heard many times. Always keep this in mind. Keep repeating, "I am going to die for the benefit of all sentient beings. The practice, the service, that I am doing and have done is for the benefit of sentient beings."

All during the day, every day, you should live with a bodhichitta motivation. Live your life to serve others. Think, "I'm here to free all sentient beings from samsara and lead them to enlightenment, bringing them happiness in this life and in all future lives and liberation from samsara."

Practicing the Five Powers

Another fundamental practice is to integrate your life practice with the five powers. This practice makes life most meaningful and beneficial for all sentient beings, and also prevents you from creating obstacles to the path. You can do other practices – sadhanas and mantras – but this is the foundation. There are five powers to be practiced in daily life, and five powers to practice at the time of death. You should know the outline of these two sets of five powers. If you are able to practice the five powers in your daily life, then you will be able to practice them at the time of death.

Meditate on the five powers at the time of death. Basically, this involves changing one's attitude into bodhichitta. Memorize and meditate on these five powers all the time; integrate your life practice with them. This should be your fundamental practice. You can also meditate on emptiness. This practice of the five powers makes us let go of what binds us to this life and to samsara; instead, we direct our life toward enlightenment. This is like untying our leg that is tied to a rock, so there is no longer anything keeping us from flying away. This is the preparation for death.

Every morning, think with complete conviction, "I am going to die today." In the afternoon, think, "I am going to die this afternoon." Then, in the evening, "I am going to die tonight." The practice of Dharma begins with preparing for death. There is no solution but to practice Dharma. Then Dharma practice becomes very pure. The thought "I am going to die this hour, this minute" brings great awareness. It is very good to think like this every day. Then, on the day that you die, you won't be shocked. This helps you to accept death.

The key thing is always to make a resolution early in the morning not to be controlled by self-cherishing thoughts, resolving that, "From now on, until death, especially today, I will never be separated from bodhichitta." The rest of the day, by putting all your effort into it, try to do all your other activities with that thought. When you collect merits each day, dedicate them to actualizing bodhichitta, both for yourself and for all sentient beings. Dedicate to be able to generate bodhichitta in this life and all future lives. Study the teachings on bodhichitta so you can see that it has great meaning in your life. Knowing the extensive benefits, you can enjoy your life practicing bodhichitta.

These are the mental thoughts for dying in the correct way; not only the correct way but the most beneficial way. These thoughts make even death – your last experience of life – beneficial for others, which is the most crucial thing.

Throughout the day, it is very good to think in this way: "The purpose of my life is not only my own happiness, not only solving my own problems. The goal of my life is to free others from suffering and to cause all the happiness – temporal and ultimate – to benefit others. I'm just one living being. My importance is nothing. How much I suffer or how much happiness I achieve is nothing. There are numberless other living beings who want happiness, who don't want suffering and who need my help. Every one of them is the source of all my past, present, and future happiness. Each of them is the most precious one in my life. How incredibly fortunate I am that I can let go of my self – from which all problems and all the undesirable things come – and instead cherish others and experience their death and all their problems for them. I can let them have all the temporal and ultimate happiness."

As you are thinking like this, meditate that you take into yourself all the suffering and death of other sentient beings in the form of black smoke. Absorb this smoke through the nose and let it destroy the egocentric self-cherishing thought at your heart. The ego becomes non-existent. If you can do this meditation, it's extremely good.

The practice of Nyung Nä, the fasting retreat with Chenrezig, is an excellent method for developing the thought of bodhichitta, of cherishing others.

The Practice of Giving and Taking (Tonglen)

The best practice is tonglen. Give your suffering, your illness, your cancer to your own self-cherishing, to your attachment, aversion, and ignorance, to your delusions. Recall *The Wheel of Sharp Weapons* and accept that your suffering, for example, your cancer, is the result of your negative karma.

There are so many sentient beings with cancer and other illnesses, so many with the potential for cancer. Think to yourself, "I

am going to die anyway, so I shall use my illness as a cause to benefit all sentient beings, to generate bodhichitta. I will receive cancer
and all sentient beings' sufferings upon myself. So many times I
have made this prayer while doing Guru Puja and now it has come
true." With that, believe strongly that one has received cancer (or
whatever other sickness or difficulty) as a result of the prayers one
has made. Dedicate not only to experience cancer on behalf of all
sentient beings but to receive enlightenment quickly. Each time
you have the thought, "I have cancer," think, "I am experiencing
it for all sentient beings." When your mind is depressed or weak,
think that the cancer is destroying your ego, your worst enemy, the
demon of selfishness. At other times, experience the cancer for
others. In this way, see your illness as the path to enlightenment,
something important to have. Your illness becomes a necessity. In
this way, you purify and cease the defilements; you use your illness
to purify the cause of your illness. Thus, the cancer or other condition that frightens the mind becomes medicine. It becomes more
powerful than the Vajrasattva mantra. Although here I am talking about one who has cancer, the practice of tonglen applies to
every difficult circumstance of our lives – suffering, pain, illness,
death. As long as we are in samsara, there is no way to be healthy
or free from suffering. It is as if we are living in a fire, so we cannot expect not to be burned and to be comfortable. But we can
practice tonglen in the face of every difficulty that we experience,
from birth to death, and make our lives and all our difficulties of
great benefit to ourselves and others.

The Power of Tonglen

Once, in a previous lifetime, Buddha was a clay-maker girl, someone of a low caste. Actually she was a girl, but for some reason
to protect her life, the child was said to be a boy. His father was
a merchant who had died on the ocean, so his mother did not
want him to follow in the same trade. She asked him first to be a
grass cutter, then asked him to take another job and then another.
Finally, he decided that he would go to sea. His mother tried to

stop him by holding on to his feet, but he kicked her head and left. Once he was at sea, he passed many islands where there were beautiful maidens, etc., but he did not stop. Then at one place he saw a man whose head was gripped by a wheel. When he saw that, he thought in his mind to take that man's suffering upon himself. The wheel that would have fallen on his own head because of the negative karma of kicking his mother was immediately lifted.

There is also the story of one of the Buddha's previous lives as a bodhisattva when he was reborn in a hell realm. At that time, the bodhisattva generated the thought of great compassion, wishing to help another man who was pulling a carriage. Because of that, the bodhisattva immediately took rebirth in Tushita pure realm.

These stories illustrate that tonglen is more powerful than Vajrasattva practice. Every time you think of experiencing suffering for others, you purify so much negative karma. External medicine does not purify this. Medicine itself cannot cure disease; the more important thing is meditation. I know many people who have cured themselves of terminal disease through meditation.

So when you find out you are going to die, put all your effort into generating bodhichitta, giving sentient beings all your happiness, merit, and possessions. Meditate that they receive all this, and it causes them to actualize the path and achieve enlightenment. Do this while generating great loving kindness, wishing them to have happiness, and wishing that you cause them to have it. Then generate compassion and take their suffering, their sickness, and especially their death. Take all these into your heart, as you breathe in, and give them to your ego in order to destroy it. Then it becomes non-existent. Give all these sufferings also to the emotional "I" that appears to really exist from its own side but is actually non-existent. It becomes completely non-existent. Try to die with this motivation. If you die with this bodhichitta thought, your death becomes a cause of your enlightenment and a cause for the enlightenment of all sentient beings. Live your life with this precious thought, which is all-fulfilling for you and all-fulfilling for all sentient beings.

Immediate Protection

As you become closer to death, you should think, "I'm experiencing death on behalf of all sentient beings." Try to die with this thought. In this way, you are dying for others. Dying with the thought of others is the best way to die. All the buddhas and bodhisattvas, all the holy beings, will admire you. It will make them so happy that you are dying with this thought; this is the best path for you to open the door to all happiness. By practicing in this way, there is no suffering, there are no difficulties at the time of death. When dying like this, there is no fear, and also no lower rebirth – in the hells, as an animal, as a hungry ghost.

The most important practice is bodhichitta, then the five powers. These provide immediate protection. Learn these things and put them into practice. Of course, you should remember the five powers every day and be ready to die on any day, because it can happen at any time. Don't wait until you have cancer or some other condition because untimely death can happen at any moment. If you think, "I will practice the five powers in the future," death might come before that. If the mind is in the practice of the five powers every day, then when an earthquake, car accident, or heavy sickness occurs, your mind is already prepared. Concerning the fear of death, this will help immediately. This is my advice to you regarding the fear of death.

Purifying with the Guru

One of the reasons that we have fear of dying is that we haven't done enough purification. So we should keep in mind bodhichitta and devotion to the Guru. Following the Guru's advice with thought and action; this is guru devotion. If any heresy or negative thoughts have arisen in your mind toward any of the teachers from whom you have received initiations or teachings – any kind of teachings, however small – the best thing to do is to generate strong compassion and strong purification with regret, do the Samayavajra recitation, and do self-initiation.

You can do the very same visualization as we do in the Vajrasattva practice, visualizing Samayavajra on the crown of your head with the nectar coming down, and then meditating on the three purifications, downward, upward, and instantaneous. It is important for us especially to purify negative karma with the Guru. If you have received a highest tantric initiation, you should do Lama Chöpa every day. You can study His Holiness's commentary to the practice (*The Union of Bliss and Emptiness*, by His Holiness the Dalai Lama, Snow Lion Pubs.). You can also do the Vajrasattva tsog practice, which has incredible benefits.

There is one monk among our students who became very ill. It seemed at that time that he had serious life obstacles. Assuming that death might happen, this monk sent me his confession. Confessing one's downfalls to the Guru is an excellent practice to lighten one's karma.

Before going to bed, if you can, do the Thirty-Five Buddhas practice by reciting their names. If you can do the practice with prostrations, that is good, and if you can recite their names three times or more, that is very good. Also, do Vajrasattva practice, reciting the mantra a minimum of twenty-one times. Do an elaborate dedication by reciting the *King of Prayers*. It is easy to recite this prayer. If you can't, then dedicate the merits to actualize bodhichitta with the prayer "By the merit of myself and others..." and do the Samantabhadra dedication, "Just as the brave Manjushri and Samantabhadra, too, realized things as they are...." Then pray to actualize Lama Tsongkhapa's stainless and complete path, which unifies sutra and tantra in one's mind, and also dedicate firmly for all the students and benefactors (of your Dharma family), and for all sentient beings to flourish (in beneficial ways) forever. If possible, dedicate after each merit you collect. If that is not possible, then dedicate in the morning after your practice, and then when you go to bed. (*See the Helpful Resources section on p. 151 for more information on these practices*).

Skillful Lam-Rim Practice and Prayers

You should do the commitments you have received from your gurus. They are there to purify your mind and for you to gain realizations. If you do Lama Chöpa in the morning, there is a lam-rim prayer that is part of it. You must concentrate well while doing this prayer. It becomes a meditation on the entire lam-rim and a very skillful means to plant seeds of the whole path in just a few minutes.

Pray to your gurus and your deity again and again, many times throughout the day, like this: "From now on, in all my future lives, may I become like them, having perfect complete wisdom, perfect complete compassion, and perfect complete power to offer numberless benefits like the sky to all sentient beings. May I become like this from now on and in all my future lifetimes." Pray like this again and again many times a day. This prayer is most important for making your life most beneficial, bringing happiness and becoming a wish-granting jewel to all living beings. That includes also your family. If there's anybody you love, this is the best way to benefit them. Try to die with this prayer in your mind.

Or else, when you die, you should hold this thought in your mind: "I'm dying on behalf of all living beings." Otherwise, you can even die with the thought of your Guru in your mind.

These practices are the best phowa at the time of death.

Preparing for Death

His Holiness the Dalai Lama says that it is difficult at the time of death to really meditate as you did in life. If during your life you couldn't meditate well, then you won't be able to meditate at death; you won't be able to hold concentration.

The essence, therefore, is to have accumulated merit and done purification in everyday life in your relationship with sentient beings; with a sincere heart, loving kindness, and compassion to have served others; and to have done the hard work to benefit them. Also, to have made offerings to the Guru Triple Gem.

Practicing the good heart, that is, bodhichitta, during your life purifies so much negative karma, even very heavy karma, and it stops you from creating more. It is negative karma that makes the mind experience fear of death, and it is bodhichitta especially that stops the immeasurable suffering and the suffering rebirths that arise later from these negative actions. You should live in morality, taking the precepts from a spiritual master or in front of holy objects.

It is very important to integrate the five powers into your life and to learn the five powers to be practiced at death. These are very special practices to achieve enlightenment quickly. They involve phowa, transference of consciousness, at the time of death into a pure land. In the pure land one receives teachings on the Vajrayana, which enable one to achieve enlightenment in one lifetime. The effectiveness of phowa depends on how well you practice the five powers at death, and this depends on how well you do the general practices (of purifying and accumulating) in life.

The lam-rim teachings explain the four ways to accumulate powerful, extensive merit. You should attempt this in everyday life while doing all the normal activities of eating, sleeping, walking, and so on, rather than doing every action with worldly desire and samsaric attachment.

Make the total dedication right now in your heart and mind, because death can come any day or minute. The moment you think this, the painful mind of attachment goes away from your heart, so your mind is total peace and happiness. It is like an apple a day keeping the doctor away!

chapter 5

Practicing the Five Powers

Introduction

Here is a technique for making your life always happy, but not the usual kind of hallucinated happiness which is excited with desire, pride, and so on. As soon as you investigate the nature of this kind of hallucinated happiness, you discover that it is only suffering. Here we are talking about real inner peace and happiness, which bring satisfaction and fulfillment, and make your life meaningful.

The technique for achieving this is the five powers – integrating the practice of the five powers into one lifetime. When you live in this practice of the five powers twenty-four hours a day, every single thing you do, whatever it may be, is only for the sake of other sentient beings, who are numberless and who want happiness and do not want suffering, just as you do. Sentient beings need your help and don't want you to harm them. Like you, they only want others to benefit and help them and don't want even the slightest harm.

When you practice the five powers, every single thing you do is only for numberless sentient beings and therefore, everything you do only becomes the cause for achieving the peerless happiness of full enlightenment. This is the greatest profit that can be achieved with this life and therefore, this practice is the most beneficial for achieving peerless happiness. It means that every single action you do, whether it is meditation and prayers or doing your job, becomes the cause of happiness for all sentient beings. Since it is the best thing for all sentient beings, naturally it is also the best thing for you. This means that you will have the best, happiest life now and also the best, happiest life in the future – like the sun shining in this world and eliminating all darkness.

Practicing this integration of the five powers into one lifetime is also the best preparation for the happiest death. It makes even the end of your life the happiest. When death comes it will be the happiest death because you have done this practice during your lifetime, and also you will find it so easy to practice the five powers near the time of death. This is the best psychology of all and the best, deepest meditation.

There are five powers to be applied during this life and also five powers to be applied at the time of death.[1] The five powers at the time of death are a mind-training transference practice for directing your mind to its new rebirth. It is mentioned in the seven point thought transformation practice:

> The Mahayana instruction for transferring consciousness
>   is only the five powers.
> Therefore, cherish this conduct!

Also, the great Tibetan enlightened holy being Panchen Losang Chökyi Gyältsen, who composed the Guru Puja,[2] mentioned in the verses at the end of the Prayer of the Common Graduated Path,[3] which deal with the graduated completion stage of the path of highest yoga tantra:

> I seek your blessings to actualize in this life the path of unity
> Of clear light and the illusory body that arises
> From placing your feet, my Savior, in the eight petals of
>   my heart
> At the very center of my central channel.
>
> Should I not have completed the points of the path at the
>   time of death,
> I seek your blessings that I may be led to a pure land
> Either through the instructions of applying the five forces
> Or by the forceful means to enlightenment, the Guru's
>   transference of mind.[4]

These verses are advising that if one does not become enlightened in this life, if one is unable to actualize the completion stage of the highest yoga tantra path, the clear light and illusory body,[5] then at the time of death one should practice phowa to transfer the consciousness.

So here is the practice of the transference of consciousness (*phowa*) from the thought transformation (*lojong*) teachings. As the great enlightened being, the Tibetan lama Pabongkha Dechen Nyingpo mentioned:

> The mind-training transference technique does not employ the sounds of HIK and PHAT but it is more profound than any other method of transference of consciousness.[6]

The First Power: the Power of the White Seed

It is explained that when you are dying you should die with the six paramitas:[7]

> When you are dying, divide your belongings into three parts: Offer the first part to the Guru Triple Gem to collect merit, use one part to make charity to sentient beings, and use one part for a party[8] and so forth.[9] To do any of these is charity.

> For morality, you should confess and abstain from the downfalls of individual liberation for oneself, generate the wishing bodhichitta and entering bodhichitta, and engage in the vows. This is morality.

> Patience: If you have a grudge from the past, offer forgiveness. If the person is not next to you, dedicate one part of your material possessions and tell the person, "I have just this much; please forgive me." If the other person is unable to accept, be patient and let there be no unhappiness in your mind.

Regarding perseverance, whatever you do, do it with joy.

The other two, concentration and wisdom, are contained in these practices.[10]

Letting Go of Material Possessions

It is extremely urgent to let go of your material possessions, including those that you have the strongest attachment towards, and also to let go of people such as your children, family members, and loved ones. It is urgent to let go of these things, to cut your clinging and attachment; in other words, to let go of desire.

In the case of material possessions, you can either let go of the objects by offering to the Guru, Buddha, Dharma, and Sangha who are the field of merit, or by making charity to sentient beings. This means that you either give the objects away now, or you at least completely dedicate them by making a clear decision to offer them to the field of merit or as charity to others, even though they will physically be given later. You can do this by writing it down in a will. But even if you make a will, at least in your heart make the offering now to the Guru, Buddha, Dharma, and Sangha. Dedicate your possessions to holy objects or give them away, making charity for specific causes and in various ways that can benefit sentient beings.

Make the total dedication right now in your heart and mind, because death can come any day or minute. The moment you think this, the painful mind of attachment goes away from your heart so your mind is total peace and happiness. It is like an apple a day keeping the doctor away!

It is easy to understand offering to the Guru. When offering to the Buddha, Dharma, and Sangha, you can just offer from your heart. The main thing here, the very point of the practice, is to let go so that you don't torture yourself with attachment. This way you give yourself satisfaction, total peace, and happiness. There are no regrets and there is no worry caused by attachment. This brings peace so that your mind is free and able to do various meditation techniques at the time of death. You can do the practices you know such as phowa. By making offerings to the Buddha, Dharma, and Sangha, you are not only letting go but also creating inconceivable merit. Why? Because all three of these objects are very powerful. Even if there is nobody around to hear you, from your heart just think, "I am offering these things to Buddha, Dharma, and Sangha," and then you stop the clinging. Having offered them, think it belongs to them; then there is no more clinging.

There are infinite ideas how to make your money, belongings, and property most satisfactory, meaningful, and beneficial, so that you are not just benefiting yourself but also benefiting sentient beings by making charity to them.

Even though material possessions, the samsaric perfections, are essenceless, still you can take essence from them. It all depends on how much your heart is open, rather than being closed by wrong views. It depends on how well you understand the law of cause and effect (karma). Understanding and faith in karma opens up skies of opportunity to be most beneficial. Most beneficial for whom? Most beneficial for other sentient beings! And if something is most beneficial for others, it is naturally also most beneficial for you.

For example, you could dedicate money, property, or whatever you have towards preserving and spreading the teachings of the Buddha. Why is dedicating resources for the teachings of the Buddha most beneficial? Because whether sentient beings are one or numberless, what they all need is happiness.

Consciousness doesn't just cease at the time of death. It is not like a lamp that goes out when the fuel is finished or a candle flame that goes out when the candle has come to an end. The body and mind are totally separate; they are two different phenomena. The body is substantial and therefore has color and form. The mind is non-substantial and has no color or shape. Formless phenomena are something quite different from the body. Some people might think that the mind is something like brain waves, but the mind is not an external object that can be perceived by the eye sense. The mind is also not an object that can be perceived by the ear sense, nor is it an object that can be perceived by the nose sense, nor is it an object that can be perceived by the tongue sense, nor is it an object that can be perceived by the body sense. The mind is not an object of the five sense consciousnesses of ordinary beings like us.[11]

The mind can be an object of the sixth consciousness, the consciousness of the mind. For example, when somebody is angry, that anger can be expressed through their facial expression, which becomes tense, not peaceful, without any softness or smiles – only wrath. By seeing that form, you judge the person to be angry. Also, when a person becomes angry, their actions may become violent and their way of speaking rude or insulting; by seeing this, your mind also understands that the person is angry.

You can only tell that the person's mind is angry by these external wrathful expressions and actions, but there are times when a person doesn't show they are angry. Their mind is angry, but because it is not revealed by taking a particular form, such as violent actions, and there is no external sign of change, unless you have clairvoyance or omniscient mind you can't tell that the person is angry.

It is the same with attachment. If one person loves somebody else but the other person cannot see any change in their face or in the actions of their body or speech, then even though in reality there is attachment and love, the other person might believe that he or she doesn't love them. Normally you see that the other person "loves me," "is angry with me" or "is attached to me" by looking at the external form and whatever change of action is manifested.

The mind is an object of the sixth consciousness either by omniscience or ordinary beings' clairvoyance. Even before buddhahood, when a great yogi has achieved the path of unification in highest tantra, the atoms of the body can function as mind and mind can function as the body. For example, the mind can manifest into form.

The teachings mention the six perfections to ripen one's own mental continuum and five types of clairvoyance to ripen that of others.

Clairvoyance of miracle power: You display miraculous powers to sentient beings by manifesting in various forms or transformations. In this way you take care of sentient beings and lead them into the Dharma.

Clairvoyance of divine eye: The ability to foresee the death, transference of consciousness, and future rebirths of yourself and others. By explaining this to the object to be subdued, sentient beings, you liberate them from nihilism.

Clairvoyance of divine ear: The ability to hear the sound of extensive profound Dharma taught by the victorious ones and their spiritual sons, the bodhisattvas, in the various pure fields of the buddhas. You explain these teachings to the object to be subdued, the sentient beings.

Clairvoyance of remembering the past: With this ability to see your and others' karmic connections in the past, you explain Dharma according to the elements, their mind, and their way of thinking. (This type of clairvoyance is common in Buddhism and other religions, such as Hinduism.)

Clairvoyance of having ceased faults: This is a quality only of arya (exalted) beings who have removed their delusions. (Delusions are called faults because they cause you to fall to the lower realms.) This is the really special clairvoyance. Of course, the clairvoyance of having ceased all delusions refers only to buddhas.

There are also the psychic powers known as the five eyes:

Flesh eye: The eye that can see not only gross but also extremely subtle form. For instance, after achieving *shiné* (calm abiding), and maybe subtle generation, you can see and even count the atoms of a mountain.

Heavenly eye: You can see death, transference, and the past lives of yourself and others.

Eye of phenomena (dharma eye): Wisdom eye that can discriminate the level of realization of the arya (exalted) beings.

Wisdom eye: Transcendental wisdom directly seeing selflessness. (This could be the wisdom that is symbolized by the "third eye.")

Buddha eye: The Buddha eye is the most perfect of the five eyes. It shines everywhere, illuminating all.

This phenomenon called mind has no form and its nature is clear and able to perceive objects.

If the mind is trained in compassion, there is no question that a person can bring much peace and happiness into their own life. They can also bring much peace and happiness to their family, neighbors, the area and country where they live, to the whole world and to numberless beings in other universes. They can bring happiness to numberless suras or worldly gods, numberless asuras, numberless hell beings, hungry ghosts, and animals. When one person's mind is trained in compassion, it can cause all these numberless beings to have happiness in all their future lives, and to have the ultimate, everlasting happiness of liberation, free forever from the entire ocean of suffering of samsara – from the oceans of suffering of the hell beings, from the oceans of suffering of the hungry ghosts, from the oceans of suffering of animals, from the oceans of suffering of human beings, from the oceans of suffering of sura beings, from the oceans of suffering of the asuras, and from the oceans of suffering of the intermediate state beings. Not only that, it can also cause peerless happiness, full enlightenment, and complete bliss for each and every single one of the numberless sentient beings.

If the mind is in the habit of transforming into negative states such as anger and self-cherishing, and the person is in a position of power and influence, they can destroy not only their family members but also the people and animals in the area or country where they live, and on this earth. Historically it has been shown that when the mind of one person with influence and power becomes negative, so many millions of people in the world can be killed. This has happened quite a number of times throughout history.

Even when the body has totally disintegrated and is completely destroyed, still the sixth consciousness, the consciousness of the mind, continues from this life to the next. This is what takes birth, either through being conceived in the mother's womb, in an egg, by heat and moisture, or spontaneously born. (This last one, "spontaneously born" I call "entering" birth; examples of this are being born on a lotus in a pure land, or the consciousness taking birth inside fruit or even a rock.) The reincarnated consciousness takes birth as one of the six types of transmigratory beings.

Because of the continuity of consciousness, the mind becomes habituated to negative self-cherishing thoughts such as anger and then it harms other beings, not only in this present life but also in future lives. This is how the mind can harm all living beings. It has been harming living beings since beginningless rebirths because it has been under the control of the self-cherishing thoughts of anger, ignorance, and attachment. As long as we don't change our mind, sentient beings will receive harm from this negative mind, from ourselves, without end.

On the other hand, if the mind becomes positive and pure, unstained by self-cherishing thoughts, unstained by anger, ignorance or attachment, and developed in compassion and wisdom, then this mind can cause the peerless, everlasting happiness of full enlightenment for every single sentient being. Such a compassionate mind becomes wish-fulfilling to all sentient beings; it brings complete happiness to every sentient being.

The cause for other sentient beings to have happiness in every future life, to receive the body of a happy transmigratory being and to experience every kind of happiness must come from their own minds. It cannot come from outside. How does it come? By their minds creating the cause of happiness, which is virtue. They have to create the virtuous action of practicing morality so that in the future they will receive the body of a happy transmigratory being. They have to create the virtuous action of practicing charity so that in the future they will have wealth. They have to create the virtuous action of practicing patience so that in the future they will have a beautiful body and be surrounded by people who perfectly support them.

By living in the morality of abstaining from gossip, for example, in future lives especially, your speech will have much power and people will pay attention to whatever you say. By gossiping, on the other hand, in future lives your speech will have no power. Even if you request other people to help you they won't listen or comply; your speech will have no power to influence or persuade others. If you engage in the non-virtuous action of telling lies, in this and so many future lives even when you try to tell the truth, people will think that you are telling lies. These are some examples.

As a result of creating the non-virtuous action of sexual misconduct in this life, either later in this life or in many future lives you will experience the negative suffering effect of being sexually abused by others. Not only that, but instead of the people around you – like your husband, wife or companions – being harmonious with you, they will be against you.

When the mind becomes habituated to these non-virtuous actions, not only do you have to experience negative suffering results, but also you have the habit to engage in these negative actions – killing, stealing, sexual misconduct, telling lies, slandering, gossiping, hurting others' minds with words, ill will, covetousness, and so forth – again in future lives. Because of your habituation with these negative actions in the past, you are driven to engage in so much negative karma in many lifetimes. If you don't change your mind, if you don't purify past negative karmas such as the ten non-virtuous actions, and if you don't create good karma by practicing morality in this life by abstaining from these negative actions, then you will experience the suffering of samsara and particularly the suffering of the lower realms – the sufferings of the hells, hungry ghosts, and animals – continuously, without end, forever.

So you can see that for each individual sentient being to experience happiness in all their future lives, to have a human rebirth and so on, all depends on the good karma they create. That means all their happiness in future lives has to come from Dharma practice, which is their own virtuous actions of body, speech, and mind. Therefore, sentient beings need to be educated. They need to learn the Dharma, the teachings of the Buddha, and they need to practice. The happiness of future lives has to come from the Dharma, from the Buddha's teachings.

Not only that, but the duration of this life is very short, whereas the need for happiness in future lives is forever – right up until one achieves liberation and enlightenment.

Sentient beings like happiness and they don't want suffering. You can understand they want the highest, longest-lasting happiness by the way they do business, looking for the greatest profit, and by the way they shop for the best quality, longest-lasting items they can afford. They may not know the four noble truths as taught by Buddha:

1. True suffering – the different types of samsaric suffering.[12]
2. True cause of suffering – delusions and karma.
3. True cessation – cessation of delusions and karma and their resultant sufferings.
4. True path – the method to achieve true cessation.

Even if sentient beings have no idea of these four noble truths, their wish is to achieve everlasting happiness and liberation; freedom forever from suffering and its causes, as reasoned above.

To achieve their wish they need to cease karma and delusions, disturbing thoughts and wrong concepts, by actualizing the five paths to liberation. First they need to see all the six realms (sura, asura, humans, animals, hungry ghosts, and hell beings, which can be categorized in three: desire, form, and formless realms) as pure suffering, extremely unbearable, like being in the center of a fire, in a nest of poisonous snakes or sitting on an iron needle, then to have complete renunciation, not finding even an instant's attraction to any samsaric pleasure.

With this total renunciation, they enter the path to liberation and actualize the five paths: path of merit, preparatory path, right-seeing path, path of meditation, and path of no-more-learning. To achieve the second path, it is necessary to have the preparatory realization of the unification of *shamatha* (calm abiding) and great insight, special concentration, just as there has to be preliminary heat before wood can catch fire.

After that is the right-seeing path, the wisdom directly perceiving emptiness, which is like a burning flame. Due to that, from here starts the path that directly ceases the defilements, intellectual concepts and delusions. Then, actualizing the path of meditation ceases the wrong concepts, the simultaneously born delusions, so that even the seeds of delusions are ceased – that is liberation: the nature of the mind totally free from disturbing thoughts and obscurations, including the seeds of delusions, so that it is impossible for delusions to rise again and create the negative karma that results in suffering experiences.

Now you can see how the teachings of Buddha show the complete path to liberation. Without them there is no way that sentient beings can achieve everlasting happiness. Not just the temporal happiness and good things of this and future lives, but freedom for ever from the oceans of samsaric suffering.

Therefore, you can see why preserving and spreading the Dharma has very deep benefit for sentient beings and is the most important, precious thing. Sentient beings need to be educated and actualize the path, particularly the Mahayana Paramitayana five paths and ten bhumis; then, by practicing the four classes of tantra, cease the defilements and subtle dualistic view in a short time, within one lifetime or just a few years; become liberated from the oceans of samsara and achieve full enlightenment, the unified state of Vajradhara, much more quickly.

The great enlightened being Pabongkha Dechen Nyingpo said that if you give away what you are attached to:

> There is nothing else – not even another person creating root merits on your behalf – that can be more helpful after your death.[13]

What happens if you don't let go of the desire that clings to your possessions? Pabongkha Dechen Nyingpo told the following stories about the shortcomings of not letting go.[14]

A fully ordained monk[15] was attached to his begging bowl and was reborn as a snake. The Buddha chased the snake into the forest and the snake got angry. The fire of the snake's anger burnt down the forest and it was reborn in the hell realms, which means the snake's consciousness transmigrated to the hells. So what happened here is that the human body of the fully ordained monk was burned by the fire of attachment and that caused him to migrate into a snake's body. The snake's body was then burned by anger, which caused the snake to migrate to the hell realms. Then the hell body was also burned by fire, so all three bodies burned in the fire.

Another person was obsessed with some gold that was hidden under the ground. This person was reborn as a snake and was forced to offer the gold to the Buddha.

If you are attached to someone else's body, or even to your own body, this can create the cause to be reborn as a worm inside that body. In ancient times in India, there was a woman's corpse lying on the ocean shore. A worm that looked like a snake lived in the corpse and would slither constantly in and out of the mouth, nose, eyes, ears, and so on. The worm was said to be the incarnation of a girl who had been attached to her own body and was always looking at herself in the mirror and then was born as this long worm, circling inside her own dead body.

There is another story of a simple monk who was extremely attached to some money. He died and was reborn as a frog that would spend its time clutching this money.

Some people find it very difficult to die due to attachment. The great enlightened being Pabongkha Dechen Nyingpo told the story of one old monk from Amdo[16] who was attached to fatty foods and was having a hard time dying. Even though he knew the meditation techniques and the tantric method of transference of consciousness, he was finding it extremely difficult and was unable to transfer his consciousness to the pure land of Buddha. A great lama from Amdo called Gungtang Jampälyang saw that this monk was having a hard time to die or transfer his consciousness, so the lama used his skillful means and said, "Make a wish to go to Tushita pure land. The fatty food there will be even better than the food we get during the holy festivals in the seventh month of each year." The monk immediately breathed his last breath.

There is some risk of these difficulties happening to us, so it is urgent and an emergency that we renounce attachment. If we don't practice letting go of attachment, desire, and so forth now, then when the time of death comes, similar things as those explained in these stories can happen to us.

One day Shariputra, Buddha's heart disciple who was excellent in wisdom, went for alms in the town. He went to a house where the old father always used to eat fish from the pool behind his house. The father had died and was reborn as a fish in the pool. The mother was attached to the house so she was reborn as the man's dog. The man's enemy had been killed for raping the man's wife. Because the enemy was so attached to her, he was reborn as her son. The son caught his father, the fish, and killed it. While he ate its meat, the dog, his mother, ate the fish bones, and so was beaten by her son. His own little son, his former enemy, was sitting on his knee.

Shariputra looked through the door of the house of this family and expressed:

He eats his father's flesh and beats his mother.
The enemy he killed sits on his knee.
A wife gnaws her husband's bones.
I laugh at the existence of samsara.[17]

This story shows that even clinging to one's own home has short-comings. This kind of thing can happen to us if we don't let go.

If we die with negative thoughts, and certainly if we die with anger, attachment, or ignorance, there is no question that we will be reborn in the lower realms - in the hells, hungry ghosts, or animals. Not only that, but these negative minds make the actual time of death so painful, and they make it very difficult for the consciousness to leave the body because there is so much fear, anger, and attachment, clinging to possessions, family members, friends, and home. Because of not wanting to be separated from these things, you can't let go, you don't want to die. You can see from this how attachment creates so much fear and worry. It tortures you and makes you suffer so much.

Attachment doesn't give you the freedom to be born in a pure land of Buddha, such as Amitabha Buddha's pure land. Once you are born in Amitabha Buddha's pure land, you will never ever be reborn in the lower realms. It is impossible. Once you are born there, you are free forever from the lower realms. And if you are able to be reborn in Heruka and Vajrayogini's Pure Land, Tharpa Kachö, you will definitely achieve enlightenment in that very life. That is a very quick way to achieve enlightenment if you are unable to be enlightened in this life, on this human body.

The negative clinging mind of attachment doesn't give you any freedom. You are like a bird whose legs are fastened to a stone by rope, tied down and unable to fly. Just like that you have no freedom.

Being unable to die with a virtuous thought, such as non-ignorance, non-anger, or non-attachment, you cannot receive even a perfect human rebirth, with the eight ripened aspects, in your next life. This kind of rebirth was highly emphasized by Lama Tsongkhapa. If you can achieve a human body with the eight ripened qualities,[18] you can be very successful in achieving realizations and can proceed on the path to liberation and full enlightenment. There can be great success in actualizing the path.

Also, if you die with the non-virtuous thoughts of anger, attachment, and ignorance, you cannot achieve a human body that has every opportunity to practice Dharma, such as by living in the four Mahayana Dharma wheels.[19] The first of these four is "abiding in a harmonious place." This means being born and living in a country or place where the Buddhadharma is existing in the form of the Mahayana teachings and particularly as tantra, the secret mantra Vajrayana teachings. It also means being born in a perfect family who are fully devoted to the Buddha, Dharma and Sangha, and who want to support your Dharma practice. And it means living in a place that doesn't cause health problems and where there are no obstacles to practice. The other three are meeting a perfect virtuous friend and being able to collect merits and make prayers.

If you die with non-virtuous thoughts, you cannot even achieve a perfect human body with the seven qualities of the higher realms,[20] that of the happy transmigratory being. Not only that, but you cannot even achieve an ordinary deva or human rebirth, besides not meeting with the Dharma.

Clinging to the body causes endless and unimaginable suffering. So you should reflect on this and be able to let go. Make your mind strong and have the courage to let go.

It says in the great saint, the bodhisattva Shantideva's teaching *Engaging in the Bodhisattva Deeds (Bodhicharyavatara)*:[21]

> By being attached to one's own body
> Even things that cause little fear give rise to great fear.
> So who would not have aversion to that body which
>   causes fear
> As one would to an enemy?

This means that self-cherishing is the cause of all fear. Since this is true, if you don't exchange yourself for others but are attached to your own body, then even small dangerous things like snakes, scorpions, and so forth, which should cause little fear, give rise to great fear because of attachment to the body. So why would any wise person not have hatred to this body as to an enemy, instead of cherishing it?

It is also the self-cherishing thought that causes you to engage in all evil deeds. It is because of cherishing the I that:[22]

> One desires to engage in the means of stopping the body
>   from being hungry, thirsty and so forth, and also to heal
>   sicknesses.
> So one kills chicken, fish, deer, and wild animals,
> And lies in wait, like a cat on the path, for those who are
>   passing on the road in order to deprive others of their
>   possessions.
>
> To gain profit and serve this body that is cherished
> One would even kill one's father and mother
> And steal the property of the Three Sublime Ones, the
>   Triple Gem –
> Actions that will make one burn in the unbearable
>   suffering hell realm.[23]
>
> Therefore, why would any learned person cherish the body
> And desire to protect and make offering to it?
> Why would one not regard this body as an enemy and
>   object of blame?[24]

So stop cherishing this body at all times and in any circumstances, even when you are happy or suffering, or at the time of death.

It is because of having a body and being attached to physical pleasures that people engage in all forms of sexual misconduct, and why those who are ordained break their root vows. Because of attachment to physical pleasure, people steal other's possessions, kill, tell lies, commit slander, use harsh speech, and so forth. Attachment to the body gives rise to the negative karma of covetousness – wanting to use another person's body for your own physical comfort and pleasure.

When somebody harms your physical comfort it can cause ill will and even heresy to arise, due to attachment to the body. One might even give up the Guru – the root of the path to enlightenment – because the mind is so attached to one's own physical needs and sensual pleasure. Attachment to the body is what causes people to engage in the negative karma of drinking alcohol, which creates the karma to be born in the heaviest hot hells and the great hells, experiencing suffering for billions and billions of years. It also gives rise to the suffering that comes from engaging in the negative karma of beating others and being beaten by others. All of this is because of having a body.

We also waste an unbelievable amount of money due to attachment to the body. There are so many things used with attachment for the body and this makes the biggest bill in our life! It also makes us waste this precious human life because so much time is spent taking care of the body. So much of this precious human life, so much precious time, is totally wasted with attachment, working to obtain everything that is needed for this body.

So reflect on this body, on what it really is – just a skeleton plastered over with different bits of flesh and muscle. Inside there are the organs, veins, blood, and other fluids; a layer of skin covers it and it is adorned by hair, nails, and teeth. In their natural state none of these things is attractive. The body is filled with filthy and smelly substances and what comes out of the body is also unappealing. Why be so attached to this body and suffer so much?[25]

Think about this and then come to the conclusion: "I will never again take this bad body, which brings me so much harm! After this life, I will never again take on a suffering body created by karma and delusion. I am going to place this mind, which has no nature, on the ultimate nature of the mind, which has no true existence – in the state of dharmakaya."

The Second Power; The Power of Intention[26]

With devotion totally give yourself up to the Triple Gem, completely relying on Buddha, Dharma, and Sangha.

Motivate very strongly again and again that you will never allow yourself to come under the control of the self-cherishing thought and never separate away from bodhichitta.

Think, "From now until I achieve enlightenment, especially up to the point of death, while I am dying, in the intermediate state, and in all future lives, I will never allow myself to come under the control of self-cherishing and I will never separate from bodhichitta!"

Think, "Particularly this year, this month and all twenty-four hours of today, I will never separate from bodhichitta!"

Motivate very strongly in this way and then you won't be separated from bodhichitta. Set the intention and make a strong dedication to be really careful for however many seconds there are from now up to the time of death. Put your full effort into this, just as someone crossing over a dangerous bridge would have to pay full attention to make sure not to fall off. This is very, very important, because no matter how many negative karmas you have created in this life, if you are able to practice at the time of death it has great benefit.

To be able to recognize the signs at the time of death and immediately and easily apply meditations – such as the tantric methods for the time of death or the thought transformation practice of the five powers – depends on having practiced every day, and especially so when you are sick. Otherwise, even if you can explain these practices with your mouth, if you have not actually attempted to do them; it won't benefit. It can't benefit at all.[27]

So think, "I will never give self-grasping, delusions, and the nearing delusions[28] any chance to arise. I will never allow my conduct of body, speech, and mind to be under the control of these obscuring, disturbing emotional thoughts.

"I will not allow myself to come under the control of self-cherishing until I achieve enlightenment, from now on until I die, and especially today. And I will never separate from bodhichitta from now until I achieve enlightenment, from now until I die, and especially today."

The Third Power; the Power of Blaming the Ego[29]

As the great bodhisattva Shantideva said in *Engaging in the Bodhisattva Deeds*:

> As long as you don't drop the fire,
> The burning won't stop.
> In the same way, as long as you don't let go of the I,
> Suffering can't be abandoned.

> Therefore, to pacify your own sufferings
> And the sufferings of others,
> Give yourself up for others
> And cherish others as yourself.[30]

And:

> If the self is not exchanged for others,
> Enlightenment cannot be achieved;
> There is no happiness even in samsara.
> Leave aside happiness in the life beyond this one;
> Even the works of this life cannot be achieved.[31]

All the problems we experience in this life, including sickness, relationship problems, and all the other problems, come from cherishing the self. All of these problems are a commentary to the teaching on the shortcomings of the self-cherishing thought. Every one of these problems comes from the self-cherishing thought; therefore, put all the blame for these on the self-cherishing thought. Self-cherishing is the root of all problems. It is the cause of all obstacles and of every other undesirable thing we experience. As it is mentioned in the teachings:[32]

However much happiness there is in the world,
All comes from cherishing others.
However much suffering there is
All comes from cherishing the self.

What more is there to say?
The childish work for themselves
And the Mighty One (Buddha) works for others...[33]

Even Buddha was once the same as us, having all the same delusions and problems. But because Buddha gave up the self and cherished others, he was able to complete the path of method and wisdom, and not only achieve liberation from all the oceans of samsaric sufferings, but also cease all the gross and subtle defilements and achieve the two kayas – *dharmakaya* and *rupakaya*. Not only that, but Buddha has shown numberless sentient beings the path to liberation and enlightenment and, through this, numberless sentient beings in this world have been liberated from all their sufferings and achieved enlightenment.

In a similar way, Buddha has also liberated numberless sentient beings in many other universes from the oceans of samsaric suffering and brought them to enlightenment. In every second, Buddha is enlightening numberless beings; effortlessly and spontaneously working for sentient beings until every one of them is brought to enlightenment. All of this is because Buddha simply changed his attitude and instead of cherishing "I," cherished others.

Think, "Because I have always been a child and never changed my attitude but only cherished myself since beginningless rebirth, I have not achieved full enlightenment, nor have I achieved liberation from samsara. Instead, I have been experiencing the oceans of general samsaric sufferings and particularly, the oceans of hell beings' sufferings, the oceans of preta beings' sufferings, the oceans of animal sufferings, the oceans of human sufferings, the oceans of sura sufferings, the oceans of asura sufferings, and the oceans of intermediate beings' sufferings numberless times since beginningless rebirth.

"It is most terrifying to think that the self-cherishing thought has made me suffer from time without beginning. It hasn't allowed me to achieve the gradual path common to the lower capable being, the gradual path common to the middle capable being, or the gradual path common to the higher capable being.[34] It hasn't allowed me to achieve any realizations, not even the realizations of guru devotion and perfect human rebirth.[35] Nor has it allowed me to achieve the realizations of the very beginning stages of the path to enlightenment (lam-rim), of death and impermanence, or karma. My mental continuum has been totally empty of attainments from beginningless rebirth.

"This self-cherishing thought is what causes me the greatest harm. It is more harmful than anything else! Not only that, but as long as the self-cherishing thought abides in my heart I will never achieve enlightenment; I will not even achieve liberation from samsara. I won't achieve any realizations of the stages of the path and instead, will experience the general sufferings of samsara and particularly the oceans of sufferings of the hell realm, the oceans of sufferings of the preta realm, the oceans of sufferings of the animal realm, the oceans of sufferings of the human realm, the oceans of sufferings of the sura realm, the oceans of sufferings of the asura realm and the oceans of sufferings of the intermediate state, over and over again without end."

There is no worse, more harmful, more frightening, or more dangerous thought than the self-cherishing thought, considering all the harm it has done in the past and all the harm it will cause in the future, without end. It is the self-cherishing thought that brings every difficulty to all the people in the world – from the beggar up to the king, prime minister, or billionaire. It brings a bad reputation, whether you are high or low. It is due to self-cherishing thought that attachment, anger, all kinds of ignorance, and other delusions arise. Then you engage in actions that harm others because your only goal is to achieve happiness for yourself. You take advantage of others by harming, cheating or deceiving them, giving them hardships and difficulties, and making them experience undesirable situations.

If you constantly follow the self-cherishing thought, as well as attachment and anger, then whatever actions you do towards others is never positive but only negative. You cause others to suffer and, as a result, receive every kind of bad reputation; you have to go to prison, you are fined, you go through court cases, you are sued and lose so much money.

Take the example of alcoholics. They waste their whole life. They are not able to practice meditation, to live righteously, or even to lead a normal person's life. They can't do their job: they harm their body and they harm their family. When their minds are out of control they start fighting and beat the family. They go crazy and even kill others and endanger their own lives. Their whole life becomes like this; very sad, very hallucinated.

It is similar with people who steal, doing it over and over again because of following the self-cherishing thought instead of practicing renunciation and contentment. They constantly make problems for themselves. Again and again they get into trouble with the police and earn a bad reputation.

Even though you don't want to suffer all these different kinds of punishment, you have to experience them again and again. Even though you don't want all these difficulties to happen, again and again you have to face them. Even if nobody else kills you, you end up killing yourself by committing suicide. When emotional problems come and you can't handle them, the easiest, immediate conclusion is to kill yourself. There is no space in your mind to think of another solution. When non-virtuous and immoral actions have been done and negative karma has been collected, then emotional problems come. At that time your luck is low, your good karma is weak and your negative karma is heavy, so it is easy to receive harm from spirits who influence your mind, to kill or think of suicide. It makes people think about jumping to their death and doing all sorts of things that normally they would never think of. It is the same with attachment and anger – when you follow the self-cherishing thought you can't control these negative minds. These are some of the shortcomings of the self-cherishing thought.

Another example is the way so many people in the world suffer from relationship problems. They experience all these different problems one after another, and again it is very clear that this is due to the shortcomings of the self-cherishing thought. All the problems that we experience in relationships are due to self-cherishing thought. It is because of self-cherishing that attachment rises, and by following it, people kill their husband, their wife, or other people.

On a larger scale, self-cherishing is the cause of all wars. War is a very clear example of self-cherishing. Self-cherishing invades one person's mind and heart, along with pride and attachment. Then that person uses their power and wealth to harm and kill many millions of people in this world. By doing so, that person collects so much unimaginable negative karma that it is difficult to see how they could ever come back to the human realm again. It is difficult to imagine how they could ever escape the lower realms and take an ordinary human rebirth again, and it is difficult to imagine the inconceivably heavy sufferings that they will have to experience for eons and eons. Not only that, but when there is a war many millions of other human beings suffer. The number of animals that suffer is even greater.

Even when Dharma practitioners make mistakes and are unable to correctly devote to the virtuous friend, this is also due to the self-cherishing thought. If you let go of the self-cherishing thought and surrender to the virtuous friend, then you can correctly devote yourself to the virtuous friend. If you follow the self-cherishing thought instead of following the virtuous friend, then the self-cherishing thought doesn't like to engage in practices or follow the advice of the virtuous friend. So it is following what the self-cherishing thought wants that makes you break the advice, give rise to heresy, anger, and negative thoughts to the virtuous friend and harm the virtuous friend. All the obstacles to practicing Dharma, generating realizations and quickly achieving liberation and enlightenment are due to the self-cherishing thought. Self-cherishing thought creates problems for you and due to self-cherishing thought, you are unable to practice and instead make mistakes with the virtuous friend.

From this, you can see very clearly the shortcomings of the self-cherishing thought. It harms the root of the path – correctly devoting to the virtuous friend – which in turn harms all the realizations up to enlightenment. Self-cherishing harms you by preventing you from being able to liberate and enlighten number-less sentient beings. In this way, it interferes with and harms the welfare of numberless sentient beings.

There are countless other ways that self-cherishing harms our Dharma practice. For example, *shamatha* or calm abiding, the higher training of concentration, is the basis for the higher train-ing of wisdom, great insight, and also the basis for achieving the arya path – the wisdom directly perceiving emptiness, which di-rectly ceases all the defilements, both the disturbing thoughts obscuration and the simultaneously-born obscuration. Without this wisdom directly perceiving emptiness one cannot achieve lib-eration, the state of everlasting happiness.

Self-cherishing thought creates obstacles for us to achieve shamatha. First of all, self-cherishing causes desire and attachment to arise towards this life. It makes us afraid of taking vows or pre-cepts, so we have no interest in them and reject them. Then, even if we do take vows, self-cherishing doesn't allow us to live purely in them. Not being able to live purely in the vows is yet another shortcoming of self-cherishing.

Since self-cherishing interferes with our practice of pure mo-rality, it harms our ability to achieve shamatha, calm abiding meditation. Once we have one-pointed concentration, we can concentrate as long as we wish because our minds are free from scattering thought and sinking thought, which are the two ob-stacles to perfect concentration. Even while we are attempting to gain calm abiding, self-cherishing doesn't allow us to be success-ful. It gives us many obstacles, many emotional thoughts, and then we are not able to continue or complete the meditation.

These obstacles, the emotional negative thoughts and particularly attachment, are all related to self-cherishing. Not only that, but great anger can arise due to the self-cherishing thought, which then turns into *rlung* disease[36] and becomes harmful. So again, you can see very clearly the shortcomings of the self-cherishing thought.

When we follow the self-cherishing thought and engage in many negative actions out of attachment, particularly the attachment that clings to this life, it obscures the mind from seeing the ultimate nature, emptiness. Self-cherishing interferes with our attempts to realize emptiness, by not allowing us to meditate and causing laziness. Then we become attached to negative activities, to the deeds of this life, actions governed by attachment, pride, and so forth. We spend a lot of time and energy on these non-virtuous actions, the works of this life, and have no interest or energy to bear hardships to practice Dharma – to do the practices of listening, reflection, and meditation. Self-cherishing thought makes a lot of excuses and brings a lot of distractions. It becomes an obstacle to learn even a single subject or listen to the Buddha's profound teachings.

When we recite even just one mala of OM MANI PÄDME HUM, self-cherishing prevents us from having a virtuous motivation at the beginning. Or if we do manage to have a virtuous attitude, particularly the motivation of bodhichitta, our minds are filled with distraction during the actual body of the recitation. There is no concentration because our mind keeps going to objects of desire and so forth. All of this is due to self-cherishing thought, seeking happiness for the self. Then at the end of the recitation there is no dedication. Even if there was some concentration or visualization during the recitation, at the end we don't dedicate, or we dedicate but we don't dedicate to achieve enlightenment for all sentient beings. Or even if we do dedicate that way, we don't seal the dedication with emptiness, so the action is done, but with ignorance. In the thought transformation teachings this is referred to as "abandoning poisonous food." When we seal the dedication of merits with emptiness, the practice of "abandoning poisonous food" is done. So you see how it is difficult to have a complete virtue with pure motivation, perfect concentration and perfect dedication. This is an example of trying to engage in just one virtue.

What makes our lives empty is the self-cherishing thought. When the self-cherishing thought is abiding in our heart there is no place for bodhichitta motivation, so there is no cause for enlightenment: the great success, the peerless happiness of enlightenment. Then all of our activities, including meditation and whatever else we do, even the normal activities of eating, sleeping, going to work, and so forth don't become even the cause to achieve liberation, freeing ourselves forever from the oceans of samsaric suffering. Our lives become totally empty and meaningless because everything is done with self-cherishing thought, which is an obstacle to achieving enlightenment.

Self-cherishing causes us to have attachment to seeking future lives' samsaric happiness, and because of that, there is no renunciation to this life's samsara. This means all the activities we do, including listening, reflection, meditation, and ordinary daily activities such as eating, sleeping, and going to work, don't become even the cause to achieve liberation for ourselves, freeing ourselves forever from the oceans of samsaric suffering. So life becomes totally empty and meaningless.

Everything we do becomes the cause of samsara. Listening, reflection, meditation, eating, walking, sleeping, going to work, whatever we do, it all becomes the cause of samsara. This means it all becomes the cause to die and be reborn and suffer all over again in one of the six realms. We have already experienced this numberless times in the past.

If you really think about this carefully, you won't be able to stand it at all. You won't be able to stand the fact that in this life you are unable to stop the continuity of reincarnation. This makes your life even more empty and meaningless.

Due to self-cherishing thought and attachment clinging to this life, which is a non-virtuous thought, whatever actions we do – whether it is listening, reflection, meditation, or the normal activities of eating, walking, sitting, and going to work – all become non-virtuous actions and bring the result of suffering. Even if there is some temporary, very short-term pleasure in this life, it is just the result of previous good karma. The condition for that pleasure to ripen in this life is an action done with attachment clinging to this life and therefore, it is non-virtuous. For example, if you steal someone else's money and use that to buy food, a house, and a car, you may receive some pleasure, but the method of attaining this is non-virtuous because of the motivation and so the future result will only be suffering. Like this, since even in one day your mind is completely preoccupied with the self-cherishing thought abiding in your heart, this precious human life becomes totally empty. It is completely empty and much more meaningless than the previous example. For weeks, months, and years your whole life becomes empty and meaningless. This is the greatest loss, the saddest thing. Then, when death suddenly comes and you look back over your life, you feel that it has been totally empty and meaningless, filled only with negative karma.

You had the most precious human life and could have achieved anything, any happiness that you wished for, any of the great meanings.[37] After this life you could have been born in a pure land of Buddha, where you can become enlightened, or at least as a bodhisattva in one of the lower realms, able to do extensive works for the benefit of sentient beings. You could have received a perfect human rebirth qualified by the eight freedoms and ten richnesses and again had the opportunity to meet the Buddhadharma – the Lesser Vehicle teachings, the Mahayana paramita teachings, and the Mahayana tantric teachings, which are so rich and incredible. You could have had the opportunity to meet all of these teachings, study them, generate all the realizations and achieve enlightenment quickly, without taking too much time. You could have received a precious human body with the seven qualities or a human body endowed with the four Mahayana Dharma wheels, not just in the next life, but for many lifetimes to come until enlightenment is achieved.

Especially, you could have received a precious human body endowed with the eight ripening qualities, a powerful body and mind, like Milarepa and those many other great yogis who achieved enlightenment in one brief lifetime. With such a powerful body and mind, one can bear hardships to practice Dharma and from that one can really have great development on the path to enlightenment. Not only that, but in future lives, as one achieves higher and higher paths, one is able to offer deeper and deeper and more extensive benefits to sentient beings. So you had the potential for all of this, but you didn't take the opportunity to use it. You didn't use it. You missed out. And all of this is due to the self-cherishing thought.

Now you can see how your whole life has become totally meaningless and empty. Not only that, but filled with negative karma. Your life has only been used to create the cause to continuously experience the general sufferings of samsara and particularly the sufferings of the lower realms.

Therefore, you should decide not to allow yourself to come under the control of the self-cherishing thought, but to kick it out immediately, cast it off, and renounce from the heart the great demon of self-cherishing.

As it is mentioned by Nagarjuna:

When a fire spark jumps on one's head or clothing, immediately one shakes it off and throws it away, not allowing it to remain there for a second. Like that, engage in the practice of immediately abandoning the self-cherishing thought the moment it arises.

In *Engaging in the Bodhisattva Deeds*, the great bodhisattva Shantideva says:

It is easy; even if I am burned, killed, or my head is cut off,
I will never surrender, whatever the circumstances,
To the enemy, the disturbing thought.[38]

The Fourth Power; the Power of Prayer

The great enlightened being Pabongkha Dechen Nyingpo explained that the fourth power, the power of prayer, doesn't mean praying to be born in a pure land of Buddha; rather it means praying to take upon yourself all the sufferings, different defilements, and negative karmas of all sentient beings, and also praying to generate bodhichitta.[39]

Make strong prayers to never fall under the control of the delusions and the self-cherishing thought. Pray: "In all circumstances – happy or suffering, good or bad – and at all times – at death, in the intermediate state and in all future lives – I will never allow myself to fall under the control of the delusions, self-grasping and the self-cherishing thought. I will never under any circumstance separate myself from bodhichitta."

Pray also: "May I be able to remember bodhichitta my whole life, at the time of death, in the intermediate state and in all future lives. May I be able to practice in order to meet again the Guru who reveals the teachings on thought transformation and bodhichitta."

You can die while meditating fully on bodhichitta or while meditating on emptiness. If you are meditating on emptiness, in emptiness there is no such thing as birth and death, so try to die with the mind in that state of emptiness. You can think that: "Death appears to be real and existing from its own side and I believe it to exist in this way, but actually this is hallucination. There is no such thing. It is totally empty."

Just keep the mind in that state.

The Fifth Power; the Power of Training

The great enlightened Pabongkha Dechen Nyingpo explained that in normal life you should keep training your mind in bodhichitta. When your mind is thoroughly habituated to bodhichitta, then at the time of death, due to the force of this mind-training you meditate on bodhichitta while trying to transfer your consciousness. Pabongkha Rinpoche explains that this is the power of training and there is nothing more than this, nothing extra.[40]

The way to transfer the consciousness by the power of the conduct of the body is to lie down in the lion position, while recollecting that the Buddha passed away to the sorrowless state in this position. It is very helpful to remember the Buddha because it plants the seed of enlightenment and immediately protects you from being born in the lower realms. Recollecting the Buddha also makes it easy not to be controlled by delusion and easy to give rise to virtuous thoughts.

Lie with your head towards the north and on your right side while resting your right cheek on your right hand. Block your right nostril with the small finger of your right hand so no breath can go through. Place your left hand over your left thigh and breathe in and out through your left nostril while doing tonglen.[41]

Even just adopting this conduct of lying down on the bed on your right side in the position of the lion, as the Buddha did when passing away, can make a big difference to the way you die. It makes it much easier for you to be reborn in a pure land of Buddha.

If you wonder how it is possible to be born in a pure land of Buddha by meditating on bodhichitta, the proof is in the story of Kadampa Geshe Chekawa.[42] Kadampa Geshe Chekawa was always praying to be born in the hell realms for sentient beings, but when he was about to pass away he asked his attendant to make offerings on the altar and said, "Today I have not been successful. I have always prayed to be born in the hell realms for sentient beings but today that is not happening. Instead the pure lands are appearing!" There is a similar story about Geshe Potowa.

There are more stories, too. In the past, a mother and her daughter were swept away by a river. They both generated a good heart and were reborn in Tushita pure land.

In the south of Tibet, in Lokha, where Milarepa built the nine-story tower and where the Kadampa geshes established hermitages and monasteries, a boat made of animal skin was overloaded and about to sink. A messenger on that boat generated a good heart and jumped into the water to save the others. He didn't die and a rainbow came from his body.

So there is no doubt that if you generate bodhichitta – even just a created bodhichitta[43] and not the actual one – you will be reborn in the best place. Kadampa Geshe Chekawa said:

> There are so many famous instructions given for transfer-ring the consciousness but none of these is greater or more wonderful than this technique.[44]

There is no more wonderful technique than this, because even if you pray to be born in the hell realms you will be born in a pure land of Buddha. So whenever experiencing dangers such as death and sickness, or whatever undesirable things happen in this life, such as having a bad reputation, receiving criticism and so forth, you must always remember to apply the thought transformation practice of taking and giving.

Furthermore, the great enlightened Pabongkha Dechen Nying-po explained that even though we think that phowa, the special tantric technique of transferring consciousness to a pure land, is a great thing, and that to recite the mantras HIK and PHAT and have the signs of having achieved phowa is very important, actu-ally if we train ourselves by reciting HIK many times without any visualization, we may still have the sign of transferring the con-sciousness at the crown, but that is due to the action of the wind and nothing to aspire to. The lojong technique of transferring the consciousness by thought transformation doesn't use the mantras HIK and PHAT, but transferring the consciousness using thought transformation, is the most profound of all the tantric techniques of consciousness transference.[45]

Even if you practice other phowa techniques you may still doubt whether it will close the door to the lower realms at the time of death, but if you practice transferring the consciousness with these five powers it is definite that you will never be reborn in a bad birth place – that is, in the lower realms.

So here, as His Holiness the Dalai Lama always mentions, the best way of dying is with bodhichitta. Dying with bodhichitta is a self-supporting death. That is the conclusion.

Afterword

This advice is for Buddhists. On the basis of this, other guidance can be put together for non-Buddhists, non-believers, or those who have never heard of Buddhism or studied it. When you are helping others who are not Buddhist, you can use this advice as a basis for explaining what to do, then choose and select from it what will be most helpful and fit that person. This is how the five powers can help.

The reason why I have elaborated on the five powers here, even though they are not elaborated upon in the teachings, is because in this advice I am only dealing with the five powers at the time of death. In the teachings, the explanation of the five powers at the time of death is preceded by the teaching on the five powers to be applied during one's lifetime. This preliminary teaching contains the subjects of bodhichitta meditation, exchanging self for others, the shortcomings of cherishing the self, and how to integrate the five powers into one's life. So if you are already familiar with these subjects there is no need to give much explanation about them here, you can just focus on the very essential points. This is why I have elaborated on the five powers here, but how people use this depends on the individual. Even though there are long explanations for some of the powers, still one has to come to the point, to the conclusion.

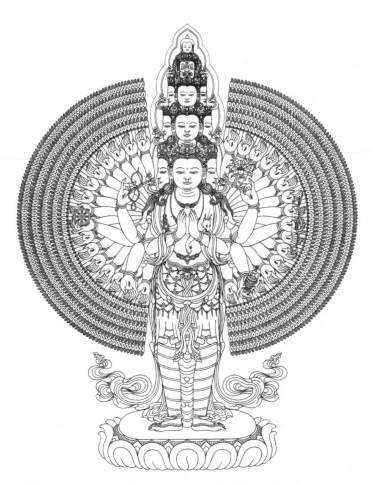

Thousand-arm Chenrezig, the Buddha of Compassion

Meditation

Taking and Giving *(Tonglen)*

Introduction

In the taking and giving meditation, we generate great compassion and take the suffering and causes of suffering of numberless other living beings upon ourselves. We use their suffering to destroy our self-cherishing thought, the source of all our problems. By generating great loving kindness, we then give other living beings everything that we have: our body, our relatives and friends, our possessions, our merit, and our happiness. We perform this practice of exchanging self for others after we have meditated on the shortcomings of self-cherishing and on the kindness of other living beings and the benefits of cherishing them. We should do the practice of taking and giving whenever we have a problem, whether it is AIDS, cancer, some other disease, the breakdown of a relationship, failure in business, or difficulty in our spiritual practice.

The taking and giving meditation is a profound and powerful practice in which we use our own pain to develop compassion for other living beings. Through this meditation, we experience our disease and all our other problems on behalf of all living beings. Doing the meditation well helps to stop our pain, and it is not uncommon for it to even heal disease. The main point of taking and giving, however, is that it purifies the causes of disease, which are in our minds.

Exchanging self for others is a brave practice, and it is far more important than visualizing light coming from healing deities or any other meditation. By taking all the suffering of others upon ourselves and giving them all our own happiness, we use our disease to generate the ultimate good heart of bodhichitta. This is the very heart of healing.

The Meditation

Taking

First generate compassion by thinking of how living beings constantly experience suffering even though they have no wish to do so, because they are ignorant of its causes, or because, although they know the causes of suffering, they are too lazy to abandon them.

Think: How wonderful it would be if all living beings could be free from all suffering and the causes of suffering, karma and delusions.

Then generate great compassion by thinking: I myself will free them from all their suffering and its causes.

As you breathe in, imagine that you take in all the suffering and causes of suffering of other living beings through your nostrils in the form of black smoke. If you have an illness or some other problem, focus first on all the numberless other beings with that same problem, then think of all the other problems experienced by living beings, as well as their causes. As you slowly breathe in the black smoke, take in all this suffering and its causes. Like plucking a thorn out of their flesh, you immediately free all the numberless living beings from all their suffering.

Next, take all the subtle obscurations from the arhats and higher bodhisattvas. There is nothing to take from the gurus and buddhas; all you can do is make offerings to them.

The black smoke comes in through your nostrils and absorbs into the self-cherishing thought in your heart, completely destroying it. Your self-cherishing, the creator of all your problems, becomes nonexistent. Like aiming a missile right on target, aim right at your self-cherishing thought, the target in this meditation.

Take from others all the undesirable environments that they experience. Breathe in through your nostrils in the form of black smoke all the undesirable places that sentient beings experience. For example, imagine that you are breathing in the red-hot burning ground of the hot hells, the ice of the cold hells, the inhospitable environments of the hungry ghosts and animals, and the dirty places of human beings. The black smoke comes in through your nostrils and down to your heart, where it absorbs into your self-cherishing thought and completely destroys it. Your self-cherishing becomes nonexistent.

Self-cherishing is based on the ignorance that holds to the concept of a truly existent I. Even though no truly existent I exists, we cherish this false I and regard it as the most precious and most important among all beings.

At the same time as your self-cherishing becomes completely non-existent, the false I that ignorance holds to be truly existent also becomes completely empty, as it is in reality. Meditate for as long as possible on this emptiness, the ultimate nature of the I.

Meditating on emptiness in this way brings powerful purification, purifying the actual cause of disease, which is the best way to cure disease.

Giving

Next, generate loving kindness by thinking that even though living beings want to be happy, they lack happiness because they are ignorant of its causes or lazy in creating them. And even if they achieve some temporary happiness, they still lack the ultimate happiness of full enlightenment.

Think: How wonderful it would be if all living beings had happiness and the causes of happiness.

Then generate great loving kindness by thinking: I myself will bring them happiness and its causes.

Visualize your body as a wish-granting jewel, which grants all the wishes of living beings. Then give everything you have to every living being. Give all your good karma of the three times and all the happiness that results from it up to enlightenment, your possessions, your family and friends, and your body, visualized as a wish-granting jewel. Also make offerings to all the enlightened beings.

Living beings receive everything that they want, including all the realizations of the path to enlightenment. Those who want a friend find a friend; those who want a Guru find a perfect Guru; those who want a job find a job; those who want a doctor find a qualified doctor; those who want medicine, find medicine. For those with incurable diseases, you become the medicine that cures them.

Since the main human problem is difficulty in finding the means of living, imagine that each human being is showered with millions of dollars from your body, which is a wish-granting jewel. You can also think that the environment becomes a pure land—the pure land of Amitabha or of the Buddha of Compassion, for example. You grant all human beings everything they want, including a pure land with perfect enjoyments. All these enjoyments cause them only to generate the path to enlightenment within their mind, and they all become enlightened.

In a similar way, give the worldly gods, the asuras and suras, everything they need, such as protective armor. They all also then become enlightened.

When you do the practice of giving to all the hell beings, completely transform their environment into a blissful pure land, with perfect enjoyments and no suffering at all. Visualize the hells as pure realms, as beautiful as possible. All the iron houses of the hell beings, which are one with fire, become jewel palaces and mandalas. All the hell beings receive everything they want and then become enlightened.

Do the same for the hungry ghosts. Transform their environment into a pure realm and give them thousands of different foods that all taste like nectar. The hungry ghosts receive everything they need, but the ultimate point is that they all become enlightened.

Since animals mainly need protection, manifest as Vajrapani or another wrathful deity to protect them from being attacked by other animals. They receive everything they want, and everything they receive becomes the cause for them to actualize the path and become enlightened.

Give also to the arhats and bodhisattvas. Give them whatever realizations they need to complete the path to enlightenment.

After everyone has become enlightened in this way, rejoice by thinking: How wonderful it is that I have enlightened every single living being.

Integrating Taking and Giving with Death

The time just prior to death is crucial, and if we can manage to use this meditation to transform our minds into bodhichitta at that time, it is better than winning a million dollars in the lottery. Rather than rejecting death as something to fear, we can use it to develop our minds in the path to enlightenment. If we cannot practice this meditation at the time of our death, we miss an incredible opportunity to benefit ourselves and other living beings.

Even when we are dying, we should try to make our death beneficial for all other living beings. At the time of our death, we should think: I prayed in the past to take upon myself the suffering of death from other living beings; I am now experiencing my death on behalf of all the other living beings who are dying now and who will have to die in the future. How wonderful it would be for all of them to be free from the suffering of death and for me alone to experience it. Let them have this ultimate happiness.

Make the place as beautiful as possible; a calm, peaceful, serene, holy environment is so important. There should be beautiful views, beautiful art, flowers, images of deities and holy beings. Flowers give a very special spiritual feeling. The point is to make a positive imprint on the person's mind. Because of being there, the person's mind is elevated, and they are not afraid of dying.

chapter 6

Caring for the Dying and the Dead

During an illness the main thing is to take care of the dying person's mind. Many others can take care of the body, but we can take care of the mind.

The most worthwhile thing to do is to inspire the person to think of others with loving kindness and compassion, to wish others to be happy and free from suffering. If a person dies with the thought of benefiting others, their mind is naturally happy and this makes their death meaningful.

You can teach the person taking-and-giving (tonglen) meditation or loving kindness meditation, according to the capacity of his or her mind. If the person has a more compassionate nature, a "brave mind," they will be able to do tonglen, taking others' suffering and giving out happiness. If the person can do tonglen, that is the best way to die, as it means dying with bodhichitta. His Holiness the Dalai Lama calls this a self-supporting death. For those who don't think others are more important than themselves, wishing others happiness and to be free of suffering is more difficult.

It is very important to know a person's mind. You can teach according to their capacity: check at the time, use your own wisdom, and judge how profound a method to present to them. It would be best if you could give the dying person some idea of the death process according to tantra: the evolution of the dissolution of the elements, the senses, the consciousness, all the way to the subtle consciousness.

For a person who has lost their capacity to understand because of coma, dementia, and so forth, there is not much possibility for them to understand. We should aim to help them attain at least a precious human rebirth. This should be our aim, not that the person must necessarily believe in karma, for example, but that they die with a positive, happy mind, with loving kindness and compassion; this is our precious gift. Our main aim in taking care of the physical body is so that we can take care of the mind, to transform their mind to the positive so that at least the person can die without anger, desire, and so forth.

You should learn various methods to benefit and calm down the mind, and to benefit now and in the future. You should get an idea of what level of method to offer each person.

If, for example, one visualizes Buddha or watches the conventional nature of mind – its clarity – other thoughts such as anger and attachment do not arise. If one is able to do this at the time of death, according to the person's mind, you can talk about the "fully enlightened being" rather than the Sanskrit "Buddha." You can talk about God if that is more skillful: a compassionate God or a loving God, or Omniscient One. Explain to the person that the nature of their mind, their heart, is completely pure; that the fully enlightened one, God, is compassionate to everyone, including them. Help them to think that their loving heart is oneness with God, that the kingdom of God is within. This frees people from guilt and anger, from their negative thoughts.

Mantra, for example, helps a person to eventually attain a higher rebirth after their positive karma is used up. Even if a person doesn't want to hear mantra, still it leaves a positive imprint on the mind. Then sooner or later that person will meet the path and have the ability to practice the teachings, to clear obscurations and attain enlightenment. Even if someone becomes angry hearing mantras and dies with an angry mind, it is still better than not hearing any mantras at all and staying peaceful. In this way, step-by-step, a person's karma will bring them to the Mahayana path and to enlightenment. Someone on the Mahayana path will attain enlightenment, while an arhat is stuck, even if the arhat starts off with the higher rebirth.

One way of thinking about this issue is to not recite mantras to a dying person if it causes the person's mind to be unhappy, to generate anger, and to be disturbed at the time of death, so that he or she will not be reborn in the lower realms. However, by leaving imprints on the person's mind, Buddha's mantras offer the benefit that the person will not be reborn in the lower realms.

Even if a person becomes angry from hearing mantras, still, in the long run, they receive benefit, because the mantras leave imprints on the mind and bring them to enlightenment. This comes just through the power of hearing the Buddha's mantras. Otherwise, although the person who is dying may have a happy mind, if you don't recite mantras, you have done nothing to cause the person to achieve enlightenment, or to save him or her from the lower realms. Even though the dying person's mind may be positive, if there is desire in the mind — for example, fear of separation from family and friends — then the person won't have a peaceful mind when dying.

A person needs a positive mind in order to have a good rebirth. A positive mind means having non-anger, non-attachment, and so forth. Only then will the result be a good rebirth. Even if a person dies with anger, Buddha's powerful words — mantras, sutras, and especially the tantric method of *jangwa* — can change their rebirth, because of their power.

You may think that to have a good rebirth, the person has to have a positive mind when dying, but the goal, what you are wishing for, is for the person to achieve enlightenment. This comes from leaving imprints on the person's mind from the power of Buddha's mantras, and so on. Even if they are temporarily reborn in the lower realms because they were annoyed by the mantras, nevertheless, because of the imprints left on the mind, they will later achieve enlightenment and liberation from samsara.

There is a story about Wusun, who was about to give teachings to 500 monks. They all would have achieved arhatship upon hearing them, but Manjushri arrived before Wusun, and gave them Mahayana teachings first. The 500 monks developed heretical thoughts toward the Dharma, and were reborn in the lower realms. Wusun went to the Buddha, and said that because Man-jushri gave them Mahayana teachings, the 500 monks were re-born in the lower realms. The Buddha answered that this was very good, and that this was an example of Manjushri's skillful means. If the 500 monks had just heard teachings on the lesser path from Wusun and achieved arhatship, they would still be there now in the state of arhatship, but because of Manjushri's skillful means, they generated heretical thoughts and took rebirth in the lower realms for a shorter time, and then they achieved enlightenment.

Creating a Conducive Environment for Dying

Make the place as beautiful as possible; a calm, peaceful, serene, holy environment is so important. There should be beautiful views, beautiful art, flowers, images of deities and holy beings. Flowers give a very special spiritual feeling. The point is to make a positive imprint on the person's mind. Because of being there, the person's mind is elevated, and they are not afraid of dying.

The advice you give the person depends on what you have been doing yourself – the lam-rim, thought transformation – what you have been practicing in daily life, beyond mere sitting meditation. In general, the Mahayana has much to offer to the dying, or to anyone with problems. Highest yoga tantra is the only system that offers a real explanation of death. The precise instructions only exist in highest yoga tantra, not in other traditions. Other tradi-tions give only general instructions; they do not provide explana-tions in terms of the subtle consciousness, winds, chakras, etc.

If one becomes accomplished at phowa and receives the signs of accomplishment, then this can be the best public service – lib-erating others and helping them at the time of death.

It is okay to ask lamas to do phowa; one can ask any Tibetan lama who is a good practitioner. The lama can do phowa wherever they are, from a distance. You will need to inform the lama which direction the head is facing.

When the Person is Dying

If you have studied the death process, you will be able to recognize the stages through which a person's consciousness is passing, what elements are absorbing, and so forth, when the person is actually dying.

It is better if the family members don't cry within hearing distance, as this creates clinging in the mind of the dying person. There are sounds to help the consciousness at the time of death, sounds that benefit, such as mantras and so on. Other than this, it is best to keep quiet and don't make any sounds. You should teach the family how to create this atmosphere.

It is okay to medicate pain in order to help the person to be able to think, but medicating for mental anguish is not advisable. Sedation of this sort before death prevents the person from exhausting negative karma. Anguish becomes fruitful if the person can experience it and finish the bad karma. It is hard to tell the difference. Often families want the patient medicated, but it is more for their own comfort than the patient's.

At death, if you can, invite members of the ordained Sangha to chant mantras nicely, in an uplifting way. When they chant like this, the person feels that nothing is more important than Amitabha Buddha. They feel protected, supported, and guided.

Chanting the names of the Thirty-five Confession Buddhas is extremely powerful (*see the companion volume to this book,* Heart Practices for Death and Dying, *available from the Foundation Store at www.fpmt.org/shop*); people can come to the room and chant together. Also, it is good to chant the very powerful mantras of the five deities normally used in jangwa puja that liberate both those dying and those already dead. These mantras also purify living beings and liberate those in the lower realms. The text *Giving Breath to the Wretched* has powerful mantras and is also good to recite (*see* Heart Practices for Death and Dying).

Place a stupa on the person's chest or let them hold it. Each time the stupa touches them, it purifies negative karma. Even if the consciousness has already left the body, there is still benefit in touching the body with the stupa. This is also good to do with babies or with people who don't understand. If the person is a non-Buddhist, say that the stupa is for peace or healing or purification. The person can visualize light rays coming from the stupa.

It is also good to have a few stupas on hand for healing or to dispel spirit harm. Also, a sheet of paper with the ten great mantras written can be put on the dying person's body (at the heart) while reciting a dedication prayer (*see p. 150*)

When the Breath has Stopped

The very first thing to do after the breath has stopped is Medicine Buddha practice. As a group or individually (and for animals as well), chant the names of the Medicine Buddhas and the mantra (*see p. 149*). Medicine Buddha made a promise that if anyone chants his name and mantra, all their prayers and wishes will succeed. The power of prayer has been accomplished by Medicine Buddha, so this practice is very powerful to make your prayers succeed. From among the ten powers, one is the power of prayer; pray as if you are the Medicine Buddha's agent, on behalf of the being who has died.

Then you can do Amitabha phowa, transference of consciousness to a pure land, followed by other practices.

Recite *Sang Chö, The Prayer of Good Deeds*, commonly known as *The King of Prayers*. At funerals, it is also good for everyone attending to read this prayer together.

You can recite the Namgyälma mantra twenty-one times, then blow on water, sesame seeds, perfume, or talcum powder, and then sprinkle that over the dead body. The Namgyälma mantra is very powerful for purifying. It is best to recite the long mantra if possible, but the short mantra can also be recited. Also, if this mantra is written on cloth or paper and placed on a mountaintop or roof where the wind can blow it, whoever is touched by the wind receives blessings and their karma is purified. Circumambulating a stupa that contains the mantra purifies all the karma to be reborn in the hot hells.

In Tibet, after the breath stops, you would not touch the body until a lama in the village did phowa; this is important. Look for signs that the consciousness has left the body: the white drop, like pus or water from the nostril, or for a woman, blood and water from the lower part. Then, before moving the body, pull the hair in the center of the crown towards the back, so that the consciousness comes out through there.

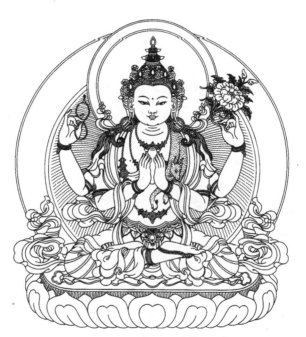

Four-arm Chenrezig, the Buddha of Compassion

The main practice to do before, during, and after death is Medicine Buddha. It is best if this practice is done near the dying person, so they can hear it being done, hear the mantra.

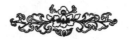

chapter 7

Essential Activities at the Death Time

This is the most essential advice given by Lama Zopa Rinpoche for the time of death. It may not be possible for everyone to do everything on the list due to lack of materials. That is all right and you shouldn't worry; just do what you can.

Before Death Essentials

If person is open to listening to mantras, any mantras are good – especially Medicine Buddha (*see p. 149*) and Compassion Buddha (*see p. 149*). There are a few that are very good, such as the mantras for pain and the sutra for pain (Recitations for Pain, *an audio CD, is available from the FPMT Foundation Store web site, www.fpmt.org/ shop*). This is very good for the dying person to listen to, especially if they are in pain (*the sutra for pain, Sutra Upon Entering the Great City of Vaishali, is also available in English in* Heart Practices for Death and Dying, *available from the Foundation Store, www.fpmt. org/shop.*).

Put holy mantras and images in a place where the dying person can see them. (The FPMT Foundation Store carries a *Card for a Dying Person*, which was personally designed by Lama Zopa Rinpoche for maximum benefit).

Place a stupa filled with the four dharmakaya relic mantras near the person. At the time of death, this stupa should be placed so it is touching the dying person's head.

The main practice to do before, during, and after death is Medicine Buddha. It is best if this practice is done near the dying person, so they can hear it being done, hear the mantra, etc. You may do the Medicine Buddha Puja or Medicine Buddha Sadhana (*included in this book on p. 135*). The simple practice is to visualize Medicine Buddha above the dying person's head. As you recite the mantra, nectar flows from the Medicine Buddha and purifies the dying person. Then make dedications for the person's future rebirth, that they may meet the Dharma, meet the perfectly qualified Mahayana teacher, practice, and become enlightened as quickly as possible. You may also dedicate that the person takes rebirth in a pure land. It is more important to focus on dedicating for the person's future rebirth rather than this life or the intermediate state. Now is the time to dedicate strongly for this person's future life to be a most precious one.

Others who care about the dying person might want to do something of benefit, and they may also do the Medicine Buddha practice themselves. When people who care about the person do this practice, it is very, very powerful.

Sponsor Medicine Buddha pujas for the dying person at a Dharma center or monastery. You may do this at Kopan Monastery in Nepal (www.kopanmonastery.org) or Land of Medicine Buddha in California (www.medicinebuddha.org), where the puja is done with extensive dedications every day.

During Death Essentials

When the death time is very close, it is best not to have anyone emotional around the dying person. Especially as the time grows very close, it is important that there is a calm and peaceful environment. No one who is crying or hanging onto the dying person should be in the room at all. This can not be stressed enough.

It is best if there are mantras playing or someone is reciting Medicine Buddha mantra in the dying person's ear (*see p. 149*).

When it seems like the person is very close to dying:

Place the sheet of mantras face down on the body, so they are touching the skin (*see p.150*).

Place a stupa so it is touching the dying person's crown.

If you have it, place Kalachakra sand on the dying person's head. (Kalachakra sand is sand from a sand mandala blessed by His Holiness the Dalai Lama). Mix the sand with butter to make it stick, and at the time of death, place it on the dying person's crown. You may also do this after the person passes away, but best is to do it before.

The main practice to do throughout this time is Medicine Buddha Puja (*for the text of this puja, see the companion volume to this book*, Heart Practices for the Dying, *available from the Foundation Store, www.fpmt.org/shop. A copy may also be downloaded from www. fpmt.org/teachers/zopa/advice/death.asp*).

When the breathing stops, no one should touch the body for as long as possible (best is seventy-two hours, but this often is not possible), even one hour (ideally the mantras and stupa would have already been placed so they are touching his body).

After Death Essentials

The first time the body is touched after the person has died, touch the crown. Tug the hair on the crown of the head so that the consciousness leaves from the crown of his head. Do a firm tug.

Recite the traditional eight prayers for the time of death. (*for the text of these prayers, see the companion volume to this book*, Heart Practices for the Dying, *available from the Foundation Store, www.fpmt. org/shop. A copy may also be downloaded from www.fpmt.org/teachers/ zopa/advice/death.asp*).

After the person passes away, again do Medicine Buddha Puja dedicated for the dying person's future rebirth. It is best to do it every day for forty-nine days, and if that is not possible, then it can be done every seventh day for forty-nine days. The last puja should have more extensive offerings, and one should recite the *King of Prayers* (one of the eight prayers for the time of death, see above).

Medicine Buddha pujas can be sponsored for the person who has died at You may do this at Kopan Monastery in Nepal (www.kopanmonastery.org) or Land of Medicine Buddha in California (www.medicinebuddha.org).

Medicine Buddha Sadhana

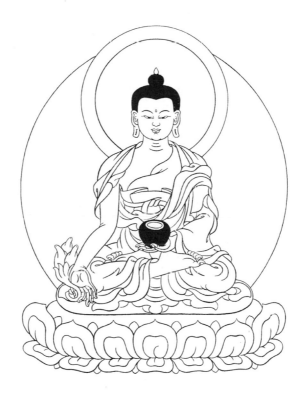

by Ngawang Losang Tempa Gyältsen

Translated by Lama Thubten Zopa Rinpoche
and prepared by Ven. Thubten Gyatso

Practice Requirements

Anyone with faith may do this practice. However, if you have not had a Medicine Buddha initiation, you may not transform into Medicine Buddha in the visualization. Instead, this visualization should be done in the space in front of you.

The Benefits of Medicine Buddha Practice

by Lama Zopa Rinpoche

The seven Medicine Buddhas, attainers of bliss, strongly prayed for the temporal and ultimate happiness of yourself and all sentient beings. They vowed that their prayers would be actualized during these degenerate times when the teachings of Shakyamuni Buddha are in decline. As the buddhas' holy speech is irrevocable, you can wholly trust in their power to quickly grant blessings to help all sentient beings in these degenerate times. If you pray to Guru Medicine Buddha, you will quickly accomplish all that you wish. Just hearing the holy name of Guru Medicine Buddha and the sound of his mantra closes the door to rebirth in the suffering lower realms. It is written in the scriptures that you should not have a two-pointed mind (doubt) with regard to these benefits.

Guru Shakyamuni Buddha said in the sutra entitled Medicine Guru Beams of Lapis Lazuli: "Kungawo, do you believe my explanation of the qualities of that tathagata [Medicine Buddha]?"

Kungawo replied to the Bhagavan: "I do not have a two-pointed mind with regard to the teachings of you, the celibate Bhagavan. Why? Because the actions of the tathagata's holy body, holy speech, and holy mind are always pure, without a single mistake."

Then Guru Shakyamuni Buddha gave this advice: "Kungawo, whoever hears the holy name of that tathagata will not fall into the evil realms of the suffering transmigratory beings."

Therefore, at the time of death, it is excellent to recite both Tathagata Medicine Buddha's holy name and his mantra in the ear of the dying person. It is extremely beneficial to recite the mantra and blow it upon meat that you are eating, or even on old bones or the dead bodies of animals or humans. This action purifies the karmic obscurations of those sentient beings. It can cause someone who has been reborn in the suffering lower realms to immediately pass away and be reborn in a pure realm or amongst happy transmigrators. At the very least, it will shorten the duration of their suffering in the lower realms. It is excellent if this is done with bodhichitta, renouncing self and cherishing others.

Also, by reciting this mantra, you will greatly enhance the power of the medicine that you are taking or giving to others. This can be done as follows:

Visualize the medicine in a bowl in front of you and above it a moon disk. Standing on the moon disk is the blue seed-syllable HUM surrounded by the syllables of the Medicine Buddha mantra in a clockwise direction. As you recite the mantra, nectars flow from all the syllables, absorbing into the medicine. The syllables and the moon then dissolve into the medicine, which becomes extremely powerful and able to cure all physical diseases and afflictions caused by spirits together with their causes, negative karma and mental obscurations of sentient beings. If you are treating a serious disease such as cancer, visualize that the medicine has the power to cure this particular disease. The stronger one's faith and the more mantras one recites, the greater will be the power of the medicine.

All existent phenomena are objects of knowing. If something is not an object of knowledge for any being, then it does not exist: an example is the 'horns of a rabbit.' All existent phenomena are included in three categories:

Objects of a valid non-deceptive consciousness, which are easily recognized, such as vase, plate, rice, flowers, and so forth;

Objects that are difficult to realize and which require reasoning to do so, such as impermanence and emptiness;

Objects that are extremely difficult to realize, such as phenomena that are only objects of knowledge of the omniscient mind. For ordinary beings, these can only be known through dependence upon scriptural authority of the Buddha.

Since the benefits of doing this sadhana are extremely difficult to recognize, they therefore belong to the third category. Only through faith in the Buddha's explanations can one realize these benefits. For those who are intellectual but somewhat thick-skulled, this explanation of the benefits and positive karma of doing the Medicine Buddha sadhana should not be discarded because it is too expansive for such a limited intelligence. If one is unable to accept this, it is better to remain indifferent rather than rejecting outright the profound teachings of the Buddha. Examine and practice this sadhana skillfully. Keep your mind steady, and you can achieve great benefits for yourself and for others without deceiving yourself.

The Benefits of Medicine Buddha Mantra

The Medicine Buddha encompasses all the buddhas. This means that when we practice the seven-limb prayer and make offerings with the seven limbs, we receive the same merit as we would if we had made offerings to all the buddhas. Similarly, when we recite the mantra of Medicine Buddha, we collect unbelievable merit just as when we offer the seven-limb practice to Medicine Buddha.

To recite the Medicine Buddha mantra brings inconceivable merit. Manjushri requested the eight tathagatas (Guru Shakyamuni Buddha and the seven Medicine Buddhas) to reveal a special mantra that would make the prayers they (the eight tathagatas) made in the past (prayers to be able to actualize the happiness of sentient beings by attaining the path to enlightenment and pacifying various problems, to be able to see all the buddhas, and for all wishes to be quickly realized) to quickly come to pass, especially for those sentient beings born in the time of the five degenerations who have small merit and who are possessed and overwhelmed by various diseases and spirit harms.

During that time, all the eight tathagatas, in one voice, taught the Medicine Buddha mantra. Therefore, if you recite the mantra every day, the buddhas and bodhisattvas will always pay attention to you, and they will guide you. Vajrapani, owner of the secrets, and the four guardians will always protect and guide you. All your negative karmas will be pacified, and you will never be born in the three lower realms. Even just hearing a recitation of the names of the eight tathagatas pacifies all diseases and spirit harms – even spirit harms that arise as a condition of disease – and all your wishes are fulfilled.

This is just a brief explanation of the benefits of the Medicine Buddha practice. This practice is especially beneficial if you are helping others, especially if you are doing healing work. It helps you to be more accurate and beneficial. You will receive much support, not only from the eight tathagatas, but from the four clairvoyant devas as well. These devas can help you to diagnose and understand the right method to heal, as they are associated with the eight tathagatas.

Medicine Buddha Sadhana

Visualization

About four inches above the crown of my head is a lotus flower. In the center of the lotus is a white moon disk and seated on the moon disk is my root Guru – the dharmakaya essence of all the buddhas – in the form of the Medicine Buddha. He is blue in color and his body radiates blue light. His right hand, in the mudra of granting sublime realizations, rests on his right knee and holds the stem of the *arura* plant between thumb and first finger. His left hand is in the mudra of concentration and holds a lapis lazuli bowl filled with nectar. He is seated in the full vajra position and is wearing the three red-colored robes of a monk. He has all the signs and qualities of a buddha.

Taking Refuge and Generating Bodhichitta

I go for refuge until I am enlightened.
To the Buddha, the Dharma, and the supreme assembly.
By my practice of giving and other perfections,
May I become a buddha in order to benefit all sentient beings. *(3x)*

The Four Immeasurable Thoughts

May all sentient beings have happiness and the causes of happiness.
May all sentient beings be free from suffering and the causes of
  suffering.

May all sentient beings never be separated from the happiness that
is without suffering.
May all sentient beings abide in equanimity, free from both attachment and hatred, holding some close and others distant.

Cultivating Special Bodhichitta

Especially for the benefit of all sentient beings, I will quickly, very
quickly, attain the precious state of perfect and complete buddhahood. For this reason I will practice the yoga method of Guru
Medicine Buddha.

Seven-Limb Prayer

I prostrate to Guru Medicine Buddha.
Each and every offering, including those actually performed and
those mentally transformed, I present to you.
I confess all non-virtuous actions accumulated since beginningless
time.
I rejoice in the virtues of both ordinary and noble beings.
As our guide I request you, O Buddha, to please abide well and
turn the wheel of Dharma until samsara ends.
All virtues, both my own and those of others, I dedicate to the
ripening of the two bodhichittas and the attainment of buddhahood for the sake of all sentient beings.

Mandala Offering (optional)

Short Mandala

This ground, anointed with perfume, strewn with flowers,
Adorned with Mount Meru, four continents, the sun and the
moon.
I imagine this as a buddha-field and offer it.
May all living beings enjoy this pure land!

Inner Mandala

The objects of my attachment, aversion and ignorance – friends, enemies and strangers – and my body, wealth, and enjoyments; without any sense of loss, I offer this collection. Please accept it with pleasure and bless me with freedom from the three poisons.

IDAM GURU RATNA MANDALAKAM NIRYATAYAMI

Prayers of Request

I beseech you, Bhagavan Medicine Guru – whose sky-colored holy body of lapis lazuli signifies omniscient wisdom and compassion as vast as limitless space – please grant me your blessings.

I beseech you, compassionate Medicine Guru – who hold in your right hand the king of medicines symbolizing your vow to help all pitiful sentient beings plagued by the 424 diseases – please grant me your blessings.

I beseech you, compassionate Medicine Guru – who hold in your left hand a bowl of nectar symbolizing your vow to give the glorious undying nectar of the Dharma that eliminates the degenerations of sickness, old age, and death – please grant me your blessings.

Visualization

Above the crown of Guru Medicine Buddha is a wish-granting jewel, which is in essence my Guru. Above that is the Buddha Delightful King of Clear Knowing (*Ngön khyen gyäl po*), whose body is coral red in color, his right hand in the mudra of bestowing sublime realizations and his left hand in the mudra of concentration. Above him is the Buddha Melodious Ocean of Proclaimed Dharma (*Chö drag gya tso yang*), with a dark pink-colored body, his right hand in the mudra of bestowing sublime realizations and his left hand in the mudra of concentration. Above him is the Buddha Supreme Glory Free from Sorrow (*Nya ngän me chog*), light pink in color with both hands in the mudra of concentration. Above him is the Buddha Stainless Excellent Gold (*Ser zang dri me*), gold in color, his right hand in the mudra of expounding the Dharma and his left hand in the mudra of concentration. Above him is the Buddha King of Melodious Sound, Brilliant Radiance of Skill, Adorned with Jewels, Moon, and Lotus (*Rin chen da wa dang pä ma rab tu gyän pa kyä pa zi ji dra yang gyi gyäl po*), yellow in color with his right hand in the mudra of expounding the Dharma and his left hand in the mudra of concentration. Above him is the Buddha Renowned Glorious King of Excellent Signs (*Tshän leg yang drag*), gold in color with his right hand in the mudra of expounding the Dharma and his left hand in the mudra of concentration.

Requests to the Medicine Buddhas

Repeat each verse seven times. After the seventh recitation as you repeat "May your vow to benefit... " the Medicine Buddha to whom the request is made absorbs into the one below.

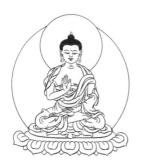

To you, Buddha Renowned Glorious King of Excellent Signs, fully realized destroyer of all defilements, fully accomplished buddha having fully realized the absolute truth of all phenomena, I prostrate, go for refuge, and make offerings. May your vow to benefit all sentient beings now ripen for myself and others. (7x)

To you, Buddha King of Melodious Sound, Brilliant Radiance of Skill, Adorned with Jewels, Moon, and Lotus, fully realized destroyer of all defilements, fully accomplished buddha who has fully realized the absolute truth of all phenomena, I prostrate, go for refuge, and make offerings. May your vow to benefit all sentient beings now ripen for myself and others. (7x)

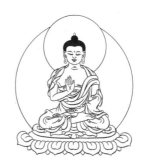

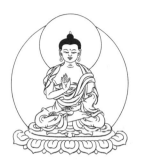

To you, Buddha Stainless Excellent Gold, Great Jewel Who Accomplishes All Vows, fully realized destroyer of all defilements, fully accomplished buddha who has fully realized the absolute truth of all phenomena, I prostrate, go for refuge, and make offerings. May your vow to benefit all sentient beings now ripen for myself and others. *(7x)*

To you, Buddha Supreme Glory Free from Sorrow, fully realized destroyer of all defilements, fully accomplished buddha who has fully realized the absolute truth of all phenomena, I prostrate, go for refuge, and make offerings. May your vow to benefit all sentient beings now ripen for myself and others. *(7x)*

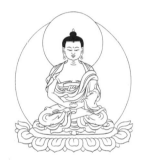

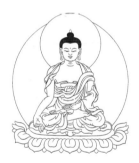

To you, Buddha Melodious Ocean of Proclaimed Dharma, fully realized destroyer of all defilements, fully accomplished buddha who has fully realized the absolute truth of all phenomena, I prostrate, go for refuge, and make offerings. May your vow to benefit all sentient beings now ripen for myself and others. *(7x)*

To you, Buddha Delightful King of Clear Knowing, Supreme Wisdom of an Ocean of Dharma, fully realized destroyer of all defilements, fully accomplished buddha who has fully realized the absolute truth of all phenomena, I prostrate, go for refuge, and make offerings. May your vow to benefit all sentient beings now ripen for myself and others. *(7x)*

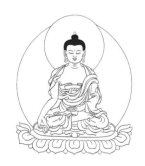

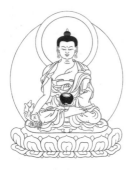

To you, Buddha Medicine Guru, King of Lapis Light, fully realized destroyer of all defilements, fully accomplished buddha who has fully realized the absolute truth of all phenomena, I prostrate, go for refuge, and make offerings. May your vow to benefit all sentient beings now ripen for myself and others. *(7x)*

Visualization

Granting your request, from the heart and holy body of the King of Medicine, Guru Medicine Buddha, infinite rays of white light pour down completely filling your body from head to toe. They purify all your diseases and afflictions due to spirits and their causes, all your negative karma and mental obscurations. In the nature of light, your body becomes as clean and clear as crystal. The light rays pour down twice more, each time filling your body with blissful clean clear light which you absorb. You are thereby transformed[47] into the holy body of Guru Medicine Buddha. At your heart appears a lotus and moon disk. Standing at the center of the moon disk, is the blue seed-syllable HUM surrounded by the syllables of the mantra. As you recite the mantra, visualize rays of light radiating out in all directions from the syllable at your heart. The light rays pervade the sentient beings of all six realms. Through your great love wishing them to have happiness, and through your great compassion wishing them to be free from all sufferings, they are purified of all diseases and afflictions due to spirits and their causes, all their negative karma and mental obscurations.

Mantra Recitation

OM NAMO BHAGAVATE BHAISHAJYE / GURU BAIDURYA / PRABHARADJAYA/TATHAGATAYA/ARHATESAMYAKSAM BUDDHAYA / TADYATHA / OM BHAISHAJYE BHAISHAJYE MAHA BHAISHAJYE [BHAISHAJYE]** / RAJA SAMUDGATE SVAHA

Short Mantra

TADYATHA / OM BHAISHAJYE BHAISHAJYE MAHA BHAISHAJYE [BHAISHAJYE] / RAJA SAMUDGATE SVAHA

[Common pronunciation: TAYATA OM BHEKANDZYE BHEKA-NDZYE MAHA BHEKANDZYE [BHEKANDZYE] RADZA SAM-UDGATE SOHA.]

Feel great joy and think:

All sentient beings are transformed into the aspect of the Medicine Buddha Guru. How wonderful that I am now able to lead all sentient beings into the Medicine Buddha's enlightenment.

Simplified Visualization

If you wish to do a shorter version instead, visualize Guru Medicine Buddha above the crown of your head and make the following prayer of request seven times:

The fully realized destroyer of all defilements, fully completed buddha having fully realized the absolute truth of all phenomena, Guru Medicine Buddha, King of Lapis Light, to you I prostrate, go for refuge, and make offerings. May your vow to benefit all sentient beings now ripen for myself and others. (7x)

As you recite the Medicine Buddha mantra, visualize as follows:

Purifying rays of light pour down from the Guru Medicine Buddha's heart and holy body, eliminating your sicknesses and afflictions due to spirits, and their causes, all your negative karma and mental obscurations. Your body is completely filled with light and becomes clean-clear like crystal. Then the rays radiate out in all directions, purifying the sicknesses and afflictions of all mother sentient beings.

After the mantra recitation visualize as follows:

The Guru Medicine Buddha melts into light and absorbs into your heart. Your mind becomes completely one with the dharmakaya, the essence of all buddhas.

Dedication

Due to these merits, may I complete the ocean-like actions of the sons of the victorious ones. May I become the holy savior, refuge, and helper for sentient beings, who have repeatedly been kind to me in past lives.

By the virtues received from attempting this practice, may all living beings who see, hear, touch, or remember me – even those who merely say my name – in that very moment be released from their miseries and experience happiness forever.*

As all sentient beings, infinite as space, are encompassed by Guru Medicine Buddha's compassion, may I too become the guide for sentient beings existing throughout all ten directions of the universe.

Because of these virtues, may I quickly become Guru Medicine Buddha and lead each and every sentient being into his enlightened realm.

* *This dedication verse includes your enemies, even when they repeat your name with anger.*

Colophon:

The Medicine Buddha Sadhana was translated by Lama Thubten Zopa Rinpoche and edited and prepared for publication by Ven. Thubten Gyatso (Adrian Feldmann) in 1982. It was first published in 1982 by Wisdom Publications. It was lightly edited and prepared for publication by the FPMT Education Department in 2001 by Ven. Constance Miller. Revised March 2002, January 2004, July 2005, January 2007.

Teaching on the Benefits of This Practice compiled from teachings given by Lama Zopa Rinpoche.

Mantras to Benefit the Dying and Dead

Mantras of the Compassion Buddha, Chenrezig (Avalokiteshvara)

NAMO RATNA TRAYAYA / NAMA ARYA JÑANA SAGARA /
VAIROCHANA VYUHA RAJAYA / TATHAGATAYA /ARHATE
SAMYAK SAMBUDDHAYA / NAMA SARVA TATHAGATABHYAH /
ARHATEBHYAH SAMYAK SAMBUDDHEBHYAH / NAMAH ARYA
AVALOKITESHVARAYA / BODHISATTVAYA / MAHASATTVAYA
MAHAKARUNIKAYA / TADYATHA / OM DHARA DHARA /
DHIRI DHIRI / DHURU DHURU /ITTI VATTE / CHALE CHALE
PRACHALE PRACHALE / KUSUME KUSUME VARE / ILI MILI /
CHITI JVALAM / APANAYE SVAHA

OM MANI PÄDME HUM

Mantras of the Medicine Buddha

OM NAMO BHAGAVATE BHAISHAJYE / GURU BAIDURYA /
PRABHA RADJAYA / TATHAGATAYA / ARHATE SAMYAKSAM
BUDDHAYA / TADYATHA / OM BHAISHAJYE BHAISHAJYE
MAHA BHAISHAJYE BHAISHAJYE / RAJA SAMUDGATE SVAHA

TADYATHA / OM BHAISHAJYE BHAISHAJYE MAHA BHAISHAJYE
BHAISHAJYE / RAJA SAMUDGATE SVAHA

[*Common pronunciation:* TAYATA OM BHEKANDZYE BHEKANDZYE
MAHA BHEKANDZYE [BHEKANDZYE] RADZA SAMUDGATE SOHA.]

The companion book to this volume, *Heart Practices for Death and Dying*, contains a plethora of other mantras, prayers, and practices to benefit the dying and dead. It is available from the Foundation Store at www.fpmt.org/shop.

These are powerful mantras to be placed on the body of one who has died. Several copies have been provided here, so that one may photocopy this page with a high quality copier (color copier recommended), cut out the mantra sheets and use them.

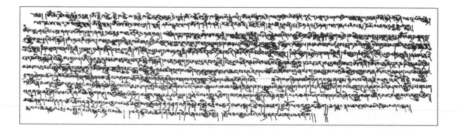

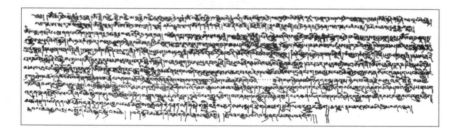

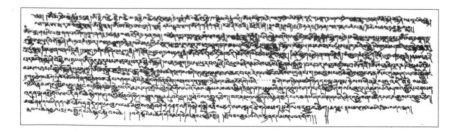

Helpful Resources

Books

Death, Intermediate State, and Rebirth by Lati Rinpoche and Jeffrey Hopkins. This fascinating book unfolds in detail the complex Tibetan Buddhist system of subtle physiology – providing a complete exposition of the channels, drops and winds which serve as foundations for consciousness. Highest Yoga Tantra simulates processes of death, intermediate states and rebirth, so it is important for the practitioner to know how we die – the stages of death and the physiological reasons behind them. Snow Lion Publications.

Mind of Clear Light: Advice on Living Well and Dying Consciously by His Holiness the XIV Dalai Lama. Using a seventeenth-century poem written by a prominent scholar-practitioner, His Holiness draws from a wide range of traditions and beliefs to explore the stages we all go through when we die. His Holiness shows us how to prepare for that time and how to enrich our time on earth, die without fear or upset, and influence the stage between this life and the next so that we may gain the best possible incarnation. As always, the ultimate goal is to advance along the path to enlightenment. *Mind of Clear Light* is an essential tool for attaining that eternal bliss. Atria Books.

Ultimate Healing: The Power of Compassion; Lama Zopa Rinpoche. We experience illness on a physical level, but in order to be healed, we must understand where true healing begins: within our hearts and minds. In *Ultimate Healing*, internationally renowned meditation master Lama Zopa Rinpoche helps us to recognize the root of illness and gives us the tools to create our future happiness. Beginning with stories of people who have recovered from disease through meditation, Rinpoche addresses the central role played by karma and by the mental habit of "labeling" in causing illness, and shows how meditation and other techniques for developing compassion and insight can eliminate the ultimate cause of all disease. Wisdom Publications.

Practice Books

Heart Practices for Death & Dying; contains essential practices to help others at the time of dying and after death. It includes a complete collection of traditional prayers and practices to be done at this crucial time. FPMT.

Medicine Buddha Puja: The Wish-Fulfilling Jewel`; Lama Zopa Rinpoche says: "It is very important that the elaborate Medicine Buddha puja be done regularly in order to benefit all. Medicine Buddha puja is also something that can be done for people who are dying, or who have already passed away, and also for individual success in all kinds of activities. This Medicine Buddha practice is extremely powerful and beneficial." FPMT.

The Preliminary Practice of Prostrations; Prostrations to the Thirty-five Confession Buddhas is one of the most powerful methods available to purify harmful actions we have done in the past. By doing this practice mindfully we can prevent unwanted sufferings from occurring in the future. In addition, this practice clears away obstacles to our practice and opens the mind to gain realizations on the path. This book contains extensive commentary by Lama Zopa Rinpoche, as well as teachings on karma, options for extended practice, and instructions on how to complete a 100,000 prostration retreat. FPMT.

The Preliminary Practice of Vajrasattva; Doing Vajrasattva retreat is not simply about reciting the mantra and saying some prayers; it is about making the practice effective for your mind, making it the quickest, most powerful way to transform your mind. Experienced meditators have advised that, in general, it is more important to put your everyday life's effort into the practice of purification - this is the way to attain spiritual realization. This practice booklet contains the short and long practice of Vajrasattva as well a Vajrasattva tsog. It also contains commentary, retreat advice, altar set-up and retreat preliminaries. FPMT.

CDs

Chants from Amitabha's Pure Land. In a hidden, secret valley in the Himalayan mountains lives a community of Tibetan Buddhist monks and nuns. Their communities were founded in the early years of the last century by Dupa Rinpoche. Dupa Rinpoche composed special prayers with heartfelt tunes that inspire and soothe the mind. *Chants from Amitabha's Pure Land* is a series of prayers requesting Amitabha Buddha to transfer the consciousness of those who have died to his pure land, a special place where all the conditions for study and practice are perfect, and enlightenment for the sake of all is achieved quickly. Sales of this CD directly benefit the monks and nuns of the Tsum valley. Chanted by the nuns of Tsum Nunnery. Daka/Dakini Productions.

Prayers for the Time of Death. In Tibetan philosophy, death is not an ending, but a transformation: the physical body is finished and the mind takes on a new form. To facilitate this transformation, death should take place in an atmosphere of calm and lightness, free of fear, with loving thoughts for our fellow beings. These beautifully chanted prayers have been chosen for their power to invoke peace and compassion in the mind of the dying person and those nearby. Chanted by the monks of Kopan Monastery. Daka/Dakini Productions.

Recitations to Alleviate Pain. Pain and disease are karmic ripenings. Often, they are the results of having harmed non-human beings in some way. The *Sutra for Entering the City of Vaishali* was given by the Buddha to Ananda specifically to pacify harmful spirits. Listening to these powerful words can help bring an end to pain. Recitations by Lama Zopa Rinpoche. FPMT.

Medicine Buddha Puja. Medicine Buddha is the manifestation of the healing energy of all enlightened beings. The seven Medicine Buddhas strongly prayed for the temporal and ultimate happiness of all sentient beings. They vowed that their prayers would be actualized during these times. Reciting the mantra purifies the karmic obscurations of all beings and greatly enhances the power of any medicine that you take. If you pray to Medicine Buddha you will accomplish quickly all that you wish. This puja is slightly more extensive than what is provided in the booklet; *Medicine Buddha, The Wish-Fulfilling Jewel*. Chanted by the monks of Kopan Monastery. Daka/Dakini Productions.

Other Helpful Materials

Liberation Card for Dying Person. This beautiful 8" x 10" color laminated card includes images and mantras that merely by seeing help a dying person to purify negative karma and be led to enlightenment. The front pictures ten mantras and ten images all especially chosen to benefit someone at the time of death. On the back of the card is a moving letter by Lama Zopa Rinpoche to assist the dying person at this most critical time. Available in English, Spanish, and Chinese. FPMT.

These materials and much more are available from the Foundation Store, www.fpmt.org/shop. Alternatively, check your local bookseller or favorite online bookstore for books listed here.

Biographies

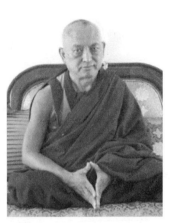

Lama Zopa Rinpoche

Lama Thubten Zopa Rinpoche was born in 1946 in the village of Thami in the Solo Khumbu region of Nepal and was recognized as the reincarnation of a great yogi, the Lawudo Lama, at the age of five. He studied with Geshe Rabten and Lama Thubten Yeshe. Soon thereafter Rinpoche and Lama Yeshe began teaching Westerners and eventually became the spiritual heads of the Foundation for the Preservation of the Mahayana Tradition (FPMT). Lama Yeshe passed away in 1984, and ever since, Lama Zopa Rinpoche has served as spiritual director of FPMT – traveling the world teaching, giving advice, sponsoring charitable projects, building holy objects, and carrying out the wishes of His Holiness the Dalai Lama. Rinpoche is the author of several books, including *Dear Lama Zopa: Radical Solutions for Transforming Problems into Happiness*, *Ultimate Healing: The Power of Compassion*, all published by Wisdom Publications.

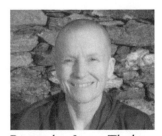

Kathleen McDonald (Venerable Sangye Khadro)

Kathleen McDonald was born in California in 1952, and took her first courses in Buddhism in Dharamsala, India in 1973. She was ordained as a Buddhist nun in 1974. She has studied Buddhism with Lama Zopa Rinpoche, Lama Thubten Yeshe, His Holiness the Dalai Lama, Geshe Ngawang Dhargyey and Geshe Jampa Tegchog, among others. At the request of her teachers, she began teaching in 1979 and has since taught in many countries around the world. She is the author of *How to Meditate*, a bestselling book published by Wisdom Publications.

Glossary

affliction See *delusion.*

aggregates (Skt: skandha) The five psycho-physical constituents that make up a sentient being: form, feeling, discriminative awareness, conditioning (compositional) factors and consciousness.

arhat (Skt; Tib: dra-chom-pa) Literally, "foe destroyer." A person who has destroyed his or her inner enemy, the delusions, and attained liberation from cyclic existence.

arya (Skt; Tib: phag-pa) Literally, noble. One who has realized the wisdom of emptiness.

Avalokiteshvara (Skt; Tib: Chenrezig) The buddha of compassion. A male meditational deity embodying fully enlightened compassion.

bardo (Tib) See intermediate state.

bhagavan (Skt; Tib: chom-dän-dä) Epithet for a buddha; sometimes translated as Lord, Blessed One and so forth. One who has destroyed (chom) all the defilements, possesses all qualities (dän) and has transcended the world (dä).

bhumi (Skt) Ground, or level, as in the ten bodhisattva levels.

bodhichitta (Skt) The altruistic intention, or determination, to reach enlightenment for the sole purpose of enlightening all sentient beings.

bodhisattva (Skt) Someone whose spiritual practice is directed toward the achievement of enlightenment. One who possesses the compassionate motivation of bodhichitta.

Buddha (Skt) A fully enlightened being. One who has removed all obscurations veiling the mind and has developed all good qualities to perfection. The first of the Three Jewels of Refuge. See also enlightenment.

Buddhadharma   The teachings of the Buddha. See also *Dharma*.

buddhahood   See *enlightenment*.

buddha nature   The clear light nature of mind possessed by all sentient beings; the potential for all sentient beings to become enlightened by removing the two obscurations: to liberation and omniscience.

Buddhist (Tib: nang-pa)   One who has taken refuge in the Three Jewels of Refuge: Buddha, Dharma and Sangha and who accepts the philosophical world view of the "four seals": that all composite phenomena are impermanent, all contaminated phenomena are in the nature of suffering, all things and events are devoid of self-existence, and nirvana is true peace.

calm abiding   See *shamatha*.

consciousness   See *mind*.

cyclic existence (Skt: samsara; Tib: khor-wa)   The six realms of conditioned existence, three lower — hell, hungry ghost (Skt: preta) and animal—and three upper — human, demigod (Skt: asura) and god (Skt: sura). It is the beginningless, recurring cycle of death and rebirth under the control of delusion and karma and fraught with suffering. It also refers to the contaminated aggregates of a sentient being.

delusion (Skt: klesha; Tib: nyön-mong)   An obscuration covering the essentially pure nature of the mind, being thereby responsible for suffering and dissatisfaction; the main delusion is ignorance, out of which grow desirous attachment, hatred, jealousy, and all the other delusions.

dependent origination   Also called dependent arising. In general, phenomena arise in dependence upon causes and conditions and are therefore empty of inherent existence; they are not self-existent because they are dependent arisings.

Dharma (Skt; Tib: chö) Spiritual teachings, particularly those of Shakyamuni Buddha. Literally, that which protects us from suffering. The Tibetan term has the literal connotation of "changing," or "bringing about transformation." The second of the Three Jewels of Refuge.

dualistic view   The ignorant view characteristic of the unenlightened mind in which all things are falsely conceived to have concrete self-existence. To such a view, the appearance of an object is mixed with the false image of its being independent or self-existent, thereby leading to further dualistic views concerning subject and object, self and other, this and that, etc.

ego   The wrong conception of the self; the mistaken belief that "I am self-existent." The fundamental ignorance that has caused us to circle through cyclic existence since beginningless time.

ego-grasping   The ignorant compulsion to regard one's self, or I, as permanent, self existent, and independent of all other phenomena.

emptiness (Skt: shunyata)   The absence of all false ideas about how things exist; specifically, the lack of the apparent independent, self-existence of phenomena. Sometimes translated as "voidness."

enlightenment (Skt: bodhi; Tib: jang-chub)   Full awakening; buddhahood. The ultimate goal of Buddhist practice, attained when all limitations have been removed from the mind and one's positive potential has been completely and perfectly realized. It is a state characterized by infinite compassion, wisdom and skill.

equanimity   Absence of the usual discrimination of sentient beings into friend, enemy and stranger, deriving from the realization that all sentient beings are equal in wanting happiness and not wanting suffering and that since beginningless time, all beings have been all things to each other. An impartial mind that serves as the basis for the development of great love, great compassion and bodhichitta.

five paths   The paths along which beings progress to liberation and enlightenment; the paths of accumulation, preparation (conjunction), seeing (insight), meditation and no more learning (beyond training).

Four Noble Truths   The subject of Buddha's first turning of the wheel of Dharma. The truths of suffering, the origin of suffering, the cessation of suffering, and the path to the cessation of suffering as seen by an arya.

graduated path (Tib: lam-rim)   A presentation of Shakyamuni Buddha's teachings in a form suitable for the step-by-step training of a disciple. The lam-rim was first formulated by the great Indian teacher Atisha (Dipankara Shrijnana, 982-1055) when he came to Tibet in 1042. See also three principal paths.

guru (Skt; Tib: lama)   A spiritual guide or teacher. One who shows a disciple the path to liberation and enlightenment. Literally, heavy with knowledge of Dharma. In tantra, one's teacher is seen as inseparable from the meditational deity and the Three Jewels of refuge.

hearer (Skt: shravaka)   A Hinayana practitioner who strives for nirvana on the basis of listening to teachings from a teacher.

Hinayana (Skt) Literally, Small, or Lesser, Vehicle. It is one of the two general divisions of Buddhism. Hinayana practitioners' motivation for following the Dharma path is principally their intense wish for personal liberation from conditioned existence, or samsara. Two types of Hinayana practitioner are identified: hearers and solitary realizers.

ignorance (Skt: avidya; Tib: ma-rig-pa)   Literally, "not seeing" that which exists, or the way in which things exist. There are basically two kinds, ignorance of karma and ignorance of ultimate truth. The fundamental delusion from which all others spring. The first of the twelve links of dependent origination.

impermanence (Tib: mi-tag-pa)   The gross and subtle levels of the transience of phenomena. The moment things and events come into existence, their disintegration has already begun.

inherent (or intrinsic) existence   What phenomena are empty of; the object of negation, or refutation. To ignorance, phenomena appear to exist independently, in and of themselves, to exist inherently.

initiation   Transmission received from a tantric master allowing a disciple to engage in the practices of a particular meditational deity. It is also referred to as an empowerment.

intermediate state (Tib: bar-do)   The state between death and rebirth.

Kadam (Tib)   The order of Tibetan Buddhism founded in the eleventh century by Atisha, Dromtönpa and their followers, the "Kadampa geshes"; the forerunner of the Gelug School, whose members are sometimes called the New Kadampas.

karma (Skt; Tib: lä)   Action; the working of cause and effect, whereby positive (virtuous) actions produce happiness and negative (non-virtuous) actions produce suffering.

lama (Tib; Skt: guru)   A spiritual guide or teacher. One who shows a disciple the path to liberation and enlightenment. Literally, heavy with knowledge of Dharma.

lam-rim (Tib)   The graduated path. A presentation of Shakyamuni Buddha's teachings in a form suitable for the step-by-step training of a disciple. See also Atisha and three principal aspects of the path.

liberation (Skt: nirvana, or moksha; Tib: nyang-dä, or thar-pa)
The state of complete freedom from samsara; the goal of a practitioner seeking his or her own escape from suffering (see also Hinayana). "Lower nirvana" is used to refer to this state of self-liberation, while "higher nirvana" refers to the supreme attainment of the full enlightenment of buddhahood. Natural nirvana (Tib: rang-zhin nyang-dä) is the fundamentally pure nature of reality, where all things and events are devoid of any inherent, intrinsic or independent reality.

lo-jong   See *mind transformation.*

mahamudra (Skt; Tib: chag-chen)   The great seal. A profound system of meditation upon the mind and the ultimate nature of reality.

Mahayana (Skt)   Literally, Great Vehicle. It is one of the two general divisions of Buddhism. Mahayana practitioners' motivation for following the Dharma path is principally their intense wish for all mother sentient beings to be liberated from conditioned existence, or samsara, and to attain the full enlightenment of buddhahood. The Mahayana has two divisions, Paramitayana (Sutrayana) and Vajrayana (Tantrayana, Mantrayana).

mantra (Skt)   Literally, mind protection. Mantras are Sanskrit syllables—usually recited in conjunction with the practice of a particular meditational deity—and embody the qualities of the deity with which they are associated.

meditation (Tib: gom)   Familiarization of the mind with a virtuous object. There are two types, placement (absorptive) and analytic (insight).

merit   Positive imprints left on the mind by virtuous, or Dharma, actions. The principal cause of happiness. Accumulation of merit, when coupled with the accumulation of wisdom, eventually results in rupakaya.

middle way   The view presented in Shakyamuni Buddha's prajña-paramita sutras and elucidated by Nagarjuna that all phenomena are dependent arisings, thereby avoiding the mistaken extremes of self-existence and non-existence, or eternalism and nihilism.

Milarepa (Tib; 1040-1123)   Tibet's great yogi, who achieved enlightenment in his lifetime under the tutelage of his guru, Marpa, who was a contemporary of Atisha. One of the founding fathers of the Kagyu School.

mind (Skt: citta; Tib: sem)   Synonymous with consciousness (Skt: vijnana; Tib: nam-she) and sentience (Skt: manas; Tib: yi). Defined as that which is "clear and knowing"; a formless entity that has the ability to perceive objects. Mind is divided into six primary consciousnesses and fifty-one mental factors.

mind transformation (Tib: lo-jong)   A genre of teaching that explains how to transform the mind from self-cherishing to cherishing others, eventually leading to the development of bodhichitta. Also known as "mind training".

Nagarjuna (Skt)   The Indian Buddhist philosopher who was born about four hundred years after the death of Shakyamuni Buddha, was said to have lived for six hundred years, and founded the Madhyamaka School of Buddhist philosophy.

nirvana (Skt; Tib: nyang-dä)   See *liberation*.

Prajñaparamita (Skt)   The perfection of wisdom. The Prajñaparamita sutras are the teachings of Shakyamuni Buddha in which the wisdom of emptiness and the path of the bodhisattva are set forth. The basis of Nagarjuna's philosophy.

preta (Skt)   Hungry ghost, or spirit. The preta realm is one of the three lower realms of cyclic existence.

puja (Skt)   Literally, offering; usually used to describe an offering ceremony.

purification   The eradication from the mind of negative imprints left by past non-virtuous actions, which would otherwise ripen into suffering. The most effective methods of purification employ the four opponent powers of regret, reliance, virtuous activity and resolve.

refuge   The door to the Dharma path. Fearing the sufferings of samsara, Buddhists take refuge in the Three Jewels with the faith that Buddha, Dharma and Sangha have the power to lead them to happiness, liberation, or enlightenment.

renunciation (Tib: nge-jung)   A heartfelt feeling of complete disgust with cyclic existence such that day and night one yearns for liberation and engages in the practices that secure it. The first of the three principal aspects of the path to enlightenment.

rinpoche (Tib)   Literally, "precious one." Epithet for an incarnate lama, that is, one who has intentionally taken rebirth in a human form to benefit sentient beings on the path to enlightenment.

root guru (Tib: tsa-wäi lama)   The teacher who has had the greatest influence upon a particular disciple's entering or following the spiritual path.

sadhana (Skt)   Method of accomplishment; the step-by-step instructions for practicing the meditations related to a particular meditational deity.

samadhi (Skt)   See single-pointed concentration.

samsara (Skt; Tib: khor- wa)   The six realms of conditioned existence, three lower—hell, hungry ghost (Skt: preta), and animal—and three upper—human, demigod (Skt: asura), and god (Skt: sura). The beginningless, recurring cycle of death and rebirth under the control of delusion and karma, fraught with suffering. Also refers to the contaminated aggregates of a sentient being.

Sangha (Skt)   Spiritual community; the third of the Three Jewels of Refuge. Absolute Sangha are those who have directly realized emptiness; relative Sangha are ordained monks and nuns.

sentient being (Tib: sem-chen)   Any unenlightened being; any being whose mind is not completely free from gross and subtle ignorance.

Shakyamuni Buddha (563-483 BC)   Fourth of the one thousand founding buddhas of this present world age. Born a prince of the Shakya clan in north India, he taught the sutra and tantra paths to liberation and enlightenment; founder of what came to be known as Buddhism. (From the Skt: buddha—"fully awake.")

shamatha (Skt; Tib: shi-nä)   Calm abiding; stabilization arisen from meditation and conjoined with special pliancy.

Shantideva   Eighth century Indian Buddhist philosopher and bodhisattva who propounded the Madhyamaka Prasangika view. Wrote the quintessential Mahayana text, A Guide to the Bodhisattva's Way of Life (Bodhicharyavatara).

shunyata (Skt)   See *emptiness.*

single-pointed concentration (Skt: samadhi)   A state of deep meditative absorption; single-pointed concentration on the actual nature of things, free from discursive thought and dualistic conceptions.

six perfections (Skt: paramita)   Charity, morality, patience, enthusiastic perseverance, concentration and wisdom.

skandha (Skt)   The five psychophysical constituents that make up a sentient being: form, feeling, discriminative awareness, conditioning (compositional) factors and consciousness.

stupa (Skt)   Buddhist reliquary objects ranging in size from huge to a few inches in height and representing the enlightened mind.

sutra (Skt)   A discourse of Shakyamuni Buddha; the pre-tantric division of Buddhist teachings stressing the cultivation of bodhichitta and the practice of the six perfections.

tantra (Skt; Tib: gyü)   Literally, thread, or continuity. The texts of the secret mantra teachings of Buddhism; often used to refer to these teachings themselves.

tathagata (Skt; Tib: de-zhin shek- pa)   Literally, one who has realized suchness; a buddha.

ten non-virtuous actions   Three of body (killing, stealing, sexual misconduct); four of speech (lying, speaking harshly, slandering and gossiping); and three of mind (covetousness, ill will and wrong views). General actions to be avoided so as not to create negative karma.

Tengyur (Tib)   The part of the Tibetan Canon that contains the Indian pandits' commentaries on the Buddha's teachings. Literally, "translation of the commentaries." It contains about 225 volumes (depending on the edition).

Three Higher Trainings   Morality (ethics), meditation (concentration) and wisdom (insight).

Three Jewels (Tib: kon-chog-sum)   The objects of refuge for a Buddhist: Buddha, Dharma and Sangha.

three principal aspects of the path   The three main divisions of the lam-rim: renunciation, bodhichitta and the right view (of emptiness).

Triple Gem   See *Three Jewels.*

Tsongkhapa, Lama Je (1357- 1417)   Founder of the Gelug tradition of Tibetan Buddhism and revitalizer of many sutra and tantra lineages and the monastic tradition in Tibet.

vows   Precepts taken on the basis of refuge at all levels of Buddhist practice. Pratimoksha precepts (vows of individual liberation) are the main vows in the Hinayana tradition and are taken by monks, nuns, and lay people; they are the basis of all other vows. Bodhisattva and tantric precepts are the main vows in the Mahayana tradition. See also Vinaya.

wisdom   Different levels of insight into the nature of reality. There are, for example, the three wisdoms of hearing, contemplation and meditation. Ultimately, there is the wisdom realizing emptiness, which frees beings from cyclic existence and eventually brings them to enlightenment. The complete and perfect accumulation of wisdom results in dharmakaya.

Notes

1. Editor: a short teaching on both of these can be found in Pabong-kha Rinpoche, *Liberation in the Palm of Your Hand*, pp. 560-563. The whole graduated path to enlightenment (*lam-rim*) is the preliminary teaching to these five powers.

2. Lama Zopa Rinpoche: The title of this text Guru Puja literally means "Pleasing the Guru." It is a practice of the most secret highest yoga tantra, which brings enlightenment in one brief lifetime of this degenerate time or even within a certain number of years.

3. Lama Zopa Rinpoche: i.e. the Paramita path.

4. Guru Puja, vv.111-112.

5. Lama Zopa Rinpoche: The clear light is the direct cause of the dharmakaya and the illusory body is the direct cause of the rupakaya.

6. *Liberation*, p. 560.

7. Lama Zopa Rinpoche translates this as the "six gone beyond." Also known as the six perfections, they are: giving, ethics, patience, perseverance, concentration, and wisdom.

8. Tib. *kye kyang*. This is an obscure word, but Lama Zopa Rinpoche thinks it means holding a party and inviting people to come, then giving things away to them.

9. Lama Zopa Rinpoche: If one is going to give things to the family it should be something that does not cause them to quarrel.

10. From the "Collection of One Hundred Teachings of Thought Transformation of the Kadampa Geshes."

11. According to Buddhist philosophy, there are five sense consciousnesses which take place on the basis of the five sense organs, those of the eye, ear, nose, tongue, body. They are not the same as the sense organs but dependent upon them. The sixth consciousness is that of the mind.

12. Lama Zopa Rinpoche: the suffering of pain, suffering of change and pervasive compounded suffering, which is the "aggregates having fault" (Tibetan: *sag che kyi püng po*), contaminated by the seed of

delusions. From this seed or imprint delusions arise, creating negative karma that makes beings reincarnate in the hell realms etc. The
continuity of the "aggregates having fault" takes rebirth in samsara,
circling from life to life.

13. *Liberation*, p. 561-2.
14. *Liberation*, pp. 562-3.
15. Lama Zopa Rinpoche: gelong, which means "virtue-beggar."
16. Lama Zopa Rinpoche: "a part of Tibet."
17. *Liberation*, p. 432.
18. The eight ripened qualities are: a long life, a handsome body, birth
    in a high family, great wealth, trustworthy speech, great power and
    fame, being born male, and being strong in mind and body.
19. These four are: living in a harmonious place, relying upon holy be-
    ings, being able to collect merit and make prayers.
20. These seven are: better family lineage, attractive physical features,
    long life, good health, good fortune, wealth and good wisdom.
21. Chapter VIII, v121.
22. Ibid, vv.122-124.
23. Lama Zopa Rinpoche: the eighth hot hell.
24. Lama Zopa Rinpoche: i.e. one should blame it.
25. This section is expanded by the editor at the suggestion of Kyabje
    Zopa Rinpoche, the main point being to contemplate the faults of
    the body in detail.
26. Lama Zopa Rinpoche also suggests the alternative use of "dedica-
    tion" or "motivation" instead of "intention" for the name of this
    power.
27. These last two paragraphs are the translation of a note written in
    Lama Zopa Rinpoche's text. Rinpoche's comment is that it could
    have been an explanation given by His Holiness the Dalai Lama.
28. Lama Zopa Rinpoche: i.e. the main delusions and twenty secondary
    delusions.
29. Lama Zopa Rinpoche: or "remorse."
30. Chapter VIII, vv.135-6
31. Ibid, vv. 131-2
32. Ibid, vv.129-30.
33. Stephen Batchelor's translation of Shantideva's *Engaging in the Bo-
    dhisattva Deeds (Guide to the Bodhisattva's Way of Life)* concludes this
    verse with the line "look at the difference between them!"

34. i.e. the "three scopes" of the graduated path to enlightenment or lamrim.

35. i.e. the very first realizations that are preliminaries to these three "scopes."

36. Tib. *rlung*: wind or air. *rlung* disease refers to an imbalance of the energy winds in the body.

37. The great meanings are the goals of the three scopes, i.e. a good rebirth, liberation, enlightenment.

38. Chapter VII, v.62. The meaning is indicating that it would be better to experience any of these terrible circumstances than to allow oneself to come under the control of the disturbing thoughts.

39. See *Liberation in the Palm of Your Hand*, p. 615.

40. *Liberation*, p. 561.

41. i.e. the practice of "taking and giving," see *Ultimate Healing*, Chapter 14.

42. This and the following stories are told by Pabongkha Rinpoche, *Liberation*, p. 563.

43. A created bodhichitta is one generated through deliberate effort; actual bodhichitta is an effortless mind-generation.

44. i.e. of the five powers.

45. This and the following paragraph cited in *Liberation*, p. 563.

46. According to Lama Zopa Rinpoche, it is "better to not use word transform, as that is like one's ordinary body becomes Buddha's body; that is not the way to meditate. Instead one's ordinary body purifies into emptiness, then the wisdom seeing emptiness takes the form of Medicine Buddha. Actually that is dharmakaya, even though in lower tantra it doesn't have the future result time dharmakaya. But actually you are visualizing yourself as Medicine Buddha, so that becomes result time deity, so that is there in kriya tantra. Your wisdom takes form of Medicine Buddha.

The point is you are not just changing the shape of your ordinary human body into shape of Buddha, like a statue of a Hindu god, and then with same material of statue you mash into shape and put on top into the shape of Buddha. You should purify into emptiness, that which is empty, not even thinking it doesn't exist, just purify into the wisdom seeing emptiness. Then label the totally new aggregates, pure aggregates, as Medicine Buddha."

References:

Pabongkha Rinpoche; *Liberation in the Palm of Your Hand* (edited by Trijang Rinpoche and translated by Michael Richards); Wisdom Publications, Boston; 1991, 1993, 1997, 2006.

Lama Zopa Rinpoche; *Ultimate Healing*: Wisdom Publications, Boston: 2001.

Index

Absorptions 65-69
AIDS 117
Amitabha 97, 120, 127, 128
Anger 16, 27, 59, 88, 91, 95, 97, 98, 104-106, 108, 124-125
Attachment 18, 27, 40, 41, 59-61, 86, 88, 90-91, 95-99, 107-108
    to the body 99-100

Bardo 16, 69-70
Bodhicharyavatara 98, 102, 111-112
Bodhichitta 20-23, 85, 101-102, 108, 109, 112, 113-115
Buddha nature 20

Cancer 11, 117, 75-76, 138
Chenrezig (Compassion Buddha) 124, 131
  mantra 149
Chekawa, Geshe 113, 114
Clairvoyance
  five types 109
  five eyes 110
Clear Light vision 66, 68
Cyclic Existence see *samsara*

Dalai Lama, His Holiness the XIV 78, 80, 115
Dark vision 67, 68-69
Death
    and Dharma practice 36, 41, 51, 58-60
    and impermanence 14, 36-37, 42-44
    assisting the dying and dead 123-134
    definite nature of 28, 50, 51-52
    fear of death 22-27, 49, 55
    nine-point meditation on 28, 49-62
    of the Buddha 55-56
    of Geshe Chekawa 113
    of yogis 68
    of Zina Rachevsky 57-58

      preparing for   73-81, 84
      process of   65-71
      remembering death   14, 23, 26, 36-42
      signs of   64-69
      uncertainty of time of   52-55
Eight Prayers   133
Elements   65-69, 89, 123, 127
Emptiness   51, 59, 75, 94, 107, 108, 112, 119
Engaging in the Bodhisattva Deeds (Bodhicharyavatara)   98, 102, 111-112
Enlightenment   13, 15, 20, 34, 36, 42, 83, 97, 100, 103, 104, 110-111

Five powers   23, 74, 78, 81, 83-115
    1. Power of the White Seed   85-111
    2. Power of Intention   101-102
    3. Power of Blaming the Ego   102-112
    4. Power of Prayer   112
    5. Power of Training   113-115
Four Noble Truths   93

Guru devotion   78, 104

Happiness   13, 17, 19, 22-23, 40, 42, 62, 66, 82, 86, 87, 90-94, 102,
      117, 119

Ignorance   26, 27, 36, 37, 53, 91, 97, 98, 104, 119
Impermanence 14-15, 33-40
    meditation on   42-43, 45-47
Intermediate State   69-70

Karma   13-14, 16-18, 21, 22, 35, 40, 43, 53, 59, 60, 65, 67, 77, 87,
      92-94, 105, 106
King of Prayers   79, 128, 134

Lam-rim   80, 81, 104, 126
Liberation   13, 15, 18, 36, 85, 90, 93-94, 103
Lion Position   113

Mantra   124-125, 149-150
    Chenrezig mantra   149
    Mantra sheet   150
    Medicine Buddha mantra   146-147, 149
Material possessions   60, 85, 86-87
Medication   127
Medicine Buddha   128, 131, 132, 133, 134, 135-148

mantras 139-140, 146-147, 149
    sadhana 141-148
Meditation 27-29, 36, 42, 45-47, 49-62, 67, 75, 77, 80, 84, 96, 101,
        105, 107-109, 117-119, 121
Milarepa 39, 111, 114
Mind 13, 39, 87-92
    at the time of death 16, 18, 26, 65, 87, 125
    body-mind relationship 15-16, 91

Pabongkha Rinpoche 85, 95, 96, 112, 113, 114
Padmasambhava 61-62
Phowa 73, 80, 81, 114, 115, 127
Prayer 112
Precious Human Rebirth 18-19, 33, 34, 93, 97, 98, 104, 110

Red vision 67

Samsara 12-13, 93, 97, 102, 109
Self-cherishing 21-23, 74, 75, 91, 99, 101-112, 117, 118
Self-grasping 100, 112
Shakyamuni Buddha 55, 59, 77, 95, 113, 126, 137, 139
Shantideva 98, 102, 111-112
Shariputra 96
Six perfections 89, 167(n)
Suffering 12, 17, 19, 23, 28, 33, 40, 41, 55-56, 60, 62, 83, 92-93

Tonglen 22, 76-77
    meditation on 117-121
Tsongkhapa 87

White vision 67

Care of Dharma Books

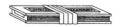

Dharma books contain the teachings of the Buddha; they have the power to protect against lower rebirth and to point the way to liberation. Therefore, they should be treated with respect – kept off the floor and places where people sit or walk – and not stepped over. They should be covered or protected for transporting and kept in a high, clean place separate from more mundane materials. Other objects should not be placed on top of Dharma books and materials. Licking the fingers to turn pages is considered bad form as well as negative karma. If it is necessary to dispose of written Dharma materials, they should be burned rather than thrown in the trash. When burning Dharma texts, it is first recite a prayer or mantra, such as OM, AH, HUM. Then, you can visualize the letters of the texts (to be burned) absorbing into the AH and the AH absorbing into you, transmitting their wisdom to your mindstream. After that, as you continue to recite OM, AH, HUM, you can burn the texts.

Lama Zopa Rinpoche has recommended that photos or images of holy beings, deities, or other holy objects not be burned. Instead, they should be placed with respect in a stupa, tree, or other high, clean place. One may put them into a small structure like a bird house and then seal the house. In this way, the holy images do not end up on the ground.

Foundation for the Preservation of the Mahayana Tradition

The Foundation for the Preservation of the Mahayana Tradition (FPMT) is a dynamic worldwide organization devoted to education and public service. Established by Lama Thubten Yeshe and Lama Zopa Rinpoche, FPMT touches the lives of beings all over the world. In the early 1970s, young Westerners inspired by the intelligence and practicality of the Buddhist approach made contact with these lamas in Nepal and the organization was born. Now encompassing over 150 Dharma centers, projects, social services and publishing houses in thirty-three countries, we continue to bring the enlightened message of compassion, wisdom, and peace to the world.

We invite you to join us in our work to develop compassion around the world! Visit our website at www.fpmt.org to find a center near you, a study program suited to your needs, practice materials, meditation supplies, sacred art, and online teachings. We offer a membership program with benefits such as Mandala magazine and discounts at the online Foundation Store. And check out some of the vast projects Lama Zopa Rinpoche has developed to preserve the Mahayana tradition and help end suffering in the world today. Lastly, never hesitate to contact us if we can be of service to you.

Foundation for the Preservation of the Mahayana Tradition
1632 SE 11th Avenue
Portland, OR 97214 USA
(503) 808-1588

www.fpmt.org

Foundation for the Preservation of the Mahayana Tradition